Medical Therapy in Urology

KT-5513-787

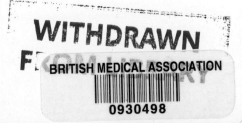

Iqbal S. Shergill · Manit Arya
Philippe Grange · Anthony R. Mundy

Medical Therapy
in Urology

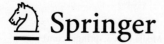

Springer

Iqbal S. Shergill
St Bartholomew's Hospital
London
UK
super_iqi@hotmail.com

Manit Arya
University College London
London
UK
manit_arya@hotmail.com

Philippe Grange
King's College Hospital
London
UK

Anthony R. Mundy
University College London
London, UK

ISBN 978-1-84882-703-5   e-ISBN 978-1-84882-704-2
DOI 10.1007/978-1-84882-704-2
Springer London Dordrecht Heidelberg New York

A catalogue record for this book is available from the British Library

Library of Congress Control Number: 2009932671

Springer is part of Springer Science+Business Media (www.springer.com)

To Maanvii Arya and Krishan Arya
who light up my life

To Navroop, Mehtaab and Partap
for their continued support and Sukhbir Khera for her
expert advice on pharmacy aspects of this textbook

Preface

The future of urology is changing from one based around surgery, to an outpatient system, concentrating mainly on medical management. Last year, in the UK, there were almost two million hospital consultations for urological symptoms and an estimated five million consultations in general practice. With such a significant proportion of care being delivered for urology, 80% of which can be managed medically, we felt that a resource should be made available to providers that will serve as a quick and useful guide to the medical management of urological disease.

The aim was to provide a fresh, practical, and concise overview of the key medical management issues every practicing clinician faces in an outpatient urology setting, on a daily basis. With these goals in mind, each chapter starts with a brief overview of the relevant anatomy/physiology and pathology of the condition in question, and then goes on to give an explanation of the drugs used, including mode of action, doses, side effects, and important interactions/contraindications. Finally, there is a brief but relevant section on review of medical literature and a clinical section on when a particular drug treatment should be used. A list of key points can be found at the end of each section.

We hope that this book will be of value to medical students, foundation year doctors, higher surgical trainees, and consultant urologists alike. Members of the multidisciplinary urology team, including nurse practitioners, continence advisors, and uro-radiologists will gain useful information and tips on medical management. Furthermore, clinicians in medical specialties and general practitioners will also be able to use it as a quick reference guide for initial medical management of most urological conditions.

This book has been an exciting and challenging project and we would like to give our heartfelt thanks to all of the chapter authors for their time and hard work. Their expertise has made our job of editing significantly easier.

London, UK

Iqbal S. Shergill
Manit Arya
Philippe Grange
Anthony R. Mundy

Contents

Contributors

Behdad Afzali
Department of Nephrology and Transplantation, MRC Centre for Transplantation, Guy's Hospital, Kings College London, London, UK

Peter Albers
Department of Urology, University Medical Center, Heinrich-Heine University Duesseldorf, Duesseldorf, Germany

Kerem B. Atalar
MRC Centre for Transplantation, King's College London, London, UK

Pierre-Marc Gilles Bouloux
Department of Endocrinology, Royal Free Hospital, London, UK

Abdul M. Chowdhury
Department of Urology, Barking, Havering and Redbridge Associated University NHS Trust, London, UK

Charlotte L. Foley
Department of Urology, Whipps Cross University Hospital, London, UK

Refik Gökmen
MRC Centre for Transplantation, Guy's Hospital, King's College London, London, UK

David J.A. Goldsmith
Guy's and St Thomas' NHS Foundation Trust, London, UK

Magnus J. Grabe
Department of Urology, Malmö University Hospital,
Malmö, Sweden

Tamsin Greenwell
Department of Urology, University College Hospital, London,
UK

Paul Irwin
Michael Heal Department of Urology, Mid-Cheshire Hospitals
NHS Foundation Trust, Leighton Hospital, Crewe, UK

Vinay Kalsi
Department of Urology, Guy's and St Thomas' Hospitals,
London, UK

Patrick F. Keane
Department of Urology, Belfast City Hospital, Belfast, UK

John D. Kelly
Department of Uro-Oncology, Division of Surgery
and Interventional Science, University College London,
London, UK

Jay Khastgir
Department of Urology, Morriston Hospital ABM University
Hospitals NHS Trust, Swansea, UK

Chi-Ying Li
Department of Urology, Princess Alexandra Hospital NHS Trust,
Harlow, UK

Brian Little
Department of Urology, The Ayr Hospital, Ayr, UK

Kim Mammen
Department of Urology, Christian Medical College and Hospital,
Ludhiana, Punjab, India

Rose McRobert
Department of Anaesthesia, The Ayr Hospital, Ayr, UK

Aza A. Mohammed
Department of Urology, The Ayr Hospital, Ayr, UK

Katie Moore
Department of Urology, Morriston Hospital ABM University Hospitals NHS Trust, Swansea, UK

Thiaga Nambirajan
Department of Urology, Belfast City Hospital, Belfast, UK

Ajay Pahuja
Department of Urology, Belfast City Hospital, Belfast, UK

Giorgio Pizzoccaro
Urologic Clinic, Milan University, San Giuseppe Hospital, Milan, Italy

Michael A. Pontari
Department of Urology, Temple University School of Medicine, Philadelphia, PA, USA

David Ralph
Department of Andrology and Urology, University College Hospital London NHS Trust, London, UK

Jose M. Reyes
Department of Urology, Temple University School of Medicine, PA, USA

William G. Robertson
Department of Physiology, Centre for Nephrology, Royal Free and University College London Medical School, London, UK

Mark A. Rochester
Department of Urology, Addenbrooke's Hospital, Hills Road, Cambridge, UK

Daniel Rottke
Department of Urology, University Medical Center Hamburg-Eppendorf, Hamburg, Germany

Wolfram E. Samlowski
Department of Medical Oncology, Nevada Cancer Institute, Las Vegas, NV, USA

Sergiy Tadtayev
Department of Urology, Lister Hospital, Stevenage, UK

Aikaterini Theodoraki
Endocrinology Department, Centre for Neuroendocrinology,
Royal Free Hospital, London, UK

Ali Thwaini
Department of Urology, Belfast City Hospital, Belfast, UK

Bryan Y. Wong
Department of Renal Cancer and Immunotherapy,
Nevada Cancer Institute, Las Vegas, NV, USA

About the Editors

Iqbal S. Shergill, BSc(Hons), MRCS(Eng), FRCS(Urol) is a senior Specialist Registrar in London. During his urology training, he has published on all aspects of urology in the medical literature as well as organized a number of practical skill courses for fellow trainees and career advice courses for medical students. He has edited four teaching textbooks and continues to be involved in teaching and training of medical/ surgical education.

Manit Arya, FRCS, FRCS(Urol) is an Honorary post-CCT Fellow in laparoscopic and minimally invasive surgery at King's College Hospital, London. He has published extensively on urology literature, as well as been an editor of five further books. He completed his higher surgical training in London and has since organized a number of local and national teaching courses both for medical students and trainees.

Philippe Grange, MD, AIH, ACCA is a Consultant Urological Surgeon and Head of Laparoscopic Surgery, at King's College Hospital, London. He has published extensively on urology literature, particularly in uro-oncology and minimally invasive surgery.

Professor Anthony R. Mundy, MS, FRCP, FRCS is Professor of Urology based at University College London Hospitals. He is also a past President of the British Association of Urological Surgeons and Civilian Consultant Urological Surgeon for the Royal Navy. He has edited numerous urology textbooks and is internationally renowned, and respected, for his significant contributions to urology.

Chapter 1
Bladder Cancer

Mark A. Rochester and John D. Kelly

Introduction

Around 70% of bladder tumors are non muscle-invasive at diagnosis and of these, 70% are stage Ta, 20% are stage T1, and 10% are carcinoma in situ (CIS). Bladder cancer is staged according to the 2002 tumor, nodes, metastases (TNM) classification approved by the Union International Contre le Cancer (Table 1.1). In this classification, papillary tumors confined to the urothelium are defined as stage Ta, whereas those invading the lamina propria are considered to be T1. By definition, CIS is confined to the urothelium and does not breach the basement membrane, but CIS has a phenotype similar to invasive disease and is associated with an aggressive outcome if left untreated. T2 tumors invade the detrusor muscle, and T3 tumors extend into the perivesical fat.

Patients with non muscle-invasive bladder cancer (NMIBC) are at significant risk of recurrence and progression. Low-grade Ta tumors progress in less than 5%. High-grade tumors pose the greatest risk for progression; Grade 3 T1 lesions carry a recurrence rate greater than 50%, and progress to muscle invasion in up to 50% of cases, especially if CIS is present

M.A. Rochester (✉)
Department of Urology, Addenbrooke's Hospital, Hills Road, Cambridge, UK

I.S. Shergill et al. (eds.), *Medical Therapy in Urology*,
DOI 10.1007/978-1-84882-704-2_1,
© Springer-Verlag London Limited 2010

TABLE 1.1.   Tumor, nodes, metastases (TNM) classification
of urinary bladder cancer.

T – Primary tumor
TX Primary tumor cannot be assessed
T0 No evidence of primary tumor
Ta Noninvasive papillary carcinoma
Tis Carcinoma in situ (CIS): "flat tumor"
T1 Tumor invades subepithelial connective tissue
T2 Tumor invades muscle
T2a Tumor invades superficial muscle (inner half)
T2b Tumor invades deep muscle (outer half)
T3 Tumor invades perivesical tissue:
T3a Microscopically
T3b Macroscopically (extravesical mass)
T4 Tumor invades any of the following: prostate, uterus, vagina, pelvic wall, abdominal wall
T4a Tumor invades prostate, uterus, or vagina
T4b Tumor invades pelvic wall or abdominal wall
N – Lymph nodes
NX Regional lymph nodes cannot be assessed
N0 No regional lymph node metastasis
N1 Metastasis in a single lymph node 2 cm or less in greatest dimension
N2 Metastasis in a single lymph node more than 2 cm but not more than 5 cm in greatest dimension, or multiple lymph nodes, none more than 5 cm in greatest dimension
N3 Metastasis in a lymph node more than 5 cm in greatest dimension
M – Distant metastasis
MX Distant metastasis cannot be assessed
M0 No distant metastasis
M1 Distant metastasis

[1,2]. Genomic alterations of cells throughout the urothelium (field change), as well as tumor cell implantation at the time of surgical resection, are responsible for recurrence and progression of disease, which necessitates a continued surveillance policy following transurethral resection of the disease. The frequency of surveillance cystoscopy is determined by the risk of recurrence and progression. An individual patient's risk depends on a number of factors, such as number, size, stage and grade of tumor, the presence of associated CIS, and the time interval between recurrences, which can be assessed

more accurately using a calculator such as that provided by the European Organisation for Research and Treatment of Cancer (EORTC), which is freely available at www.eortc.be/tools/bladdercalculator). To reduce recurrence and progression, adjuvant intravesical chemotherapy and immunotherapy, as well as novel approaches are used, and these will be discussed in this chapter.

The difference in the biological behavior of low- and high-grade urothelial carcinomas are proposed to be a consequence of separate molecular pathways, in which distinct genomic alterations are acquired during the development of the disease. Low-grade tumors harbor relatively few chromosomal abnormalities, but high-grade tumors may have numerous chromosomal changes [3]. Alterations have been mapped for high- and low-grade cancers; they are, to a degree, unique, which supports the concept that high-grade and low-grade cancers may be considered as different diseases. For the clinical management of NMIBC, it is worth considering that all G3 tumors, regardless of the stage, follow an aggressive course and, if left untreated, will progress.

Medical Therapies in Bladder Cancer

Table 1.2 summarizes the drugs used for intravesical therapy in NMIBC.

Intravesical Mitomycin Chemotherapy

Intravesical chemotherapy is used immediately postoperatively to kill free-floating cells before implantation can occur. A single dose of mitomycin, for example, administered within 6 h reduces recurrence rates more than when given at 24 h, underlining the importance of early postoperative intravesical therapy. Attempts have been made to improve on the action of intravesical chemotherapy through optimizing urine pH, volume, and bladder dwell time [4].

Mitomycin was developed in the 1970s and is commonly used in intravesical chemotherapy. It is an antitumor antibiotic

TABLE 1.2. Intravesical medical therapies for non muscle-invasive bladder cancer (NMIBC).

Intravesical therapy	Mode of action	Dose	Main side effects	Important interactions and contraindications
Mitomycin	DNA alkylating agent	40 mg in 40 ml sterile water	Skin rash, storage LUTS, bladder calcifications, and myelosuppression	Contraindicated in bladder perforation, previous reaction, Thrombocytopenia and coagulation disorder, or an increase in bleeding tendency due to other causes
Epirubicin	Topoisomerase II inhibitor	80 mg in 40 ml sterile water	Storage LUTS, systemic administration is minimal, but can be associated with myelosuppression, cardiomyopathy, congestive heart failure, and arrythmias	Contraindicated in UTI, bladder inflammation and bladder perforation
Doxorubicin	Topoisomerase II inhibitor	50 mg in 50 ml saline	Chemical cystitis, decreased bladder capacity, hematuria, fever, and allergy	Contraindicated in UTI, bladder inflammation and bladder perforation
Valrubicin	Topoisomerase II inhibitor	800 mg in 75 ml saline	chemical cystitis, decreased bladder capacity, hematuria, fever, and allergy	Contraindicated in UTI, bladder inflammation and bladder perforation

Thiotepa	DNA alkylating agent	60 mg of thiotepa in 30–60 ml saline	Fatigue, weakness, hypersensitivity, contact dermatitis, nausea, vomiting, dysuria, urinary retention	Weekly blood and platelet counts are recommended during therapy and for at least 3 weeks after therapy has been discontinued due to risk of bone marrow suppression. Avoid other alkylating agents and other bone marrow suppressants
BCG	Induces a non-specific, cytokine-mediated immune response to foreign protein	81 bmg in 50 ml saline	Dysuria, storage LUTS, hematuria, suprapubic pain, incontinence, UTI, flu-like symptoms, fever, malaise, nausea/vomiting, myalgia, allergic reaction	Contraindicated in immunosuppressed patients positive HIV serology and in patients receiving steroids at immunosuppressive therapies; concurrent febrile illness, UTI, pregnant/lactating women or gross hematuria. In addition, fourteen days should elapse before BCG is administered following biopsy, TUR, or traumatic catheterization.

acting through the inhibition of DNA synthesis. The UK Medical Research Council study BS06 confirmed that a single instillation of mitomycin administered postoperatively was effective in reducing the recurrence of NMIBC [5]. This multicentre randomized trial determined the role of one and five instillations of mitomycin in the treatment of newly diagnosed NMIBC. Following Trans-urethral resection bladder tumour (TURBT), 502 patients were randomized into one of three treatment arms: no further treatment, one instillation of mitomycin at resection, and one instillation at resection and at 3-month intervals for 1 year (five instillations). After a median follow-up of 7 years, one and five instillations of mitomycin resulted in decreased recurrence rates and increased recurrence-free interval. The benefit of mitomycin was observed in all risk groups.

This was subsequently confirmed by a meta-analysis of seven randomized trials totaling 1,476 patients with a median follow-up of 3.4 years, which reported that 36.7% of the patients receiving one postoperative instillation had tumor recurrence when compared with 48.4% with transurethral resection alone, a decrease of 39% in the odds of recurrence with chemotherapy [6]. One recent randomized trial has questioned the benefit of this approach for all patients. Gudjonsson et al. randomized 305 patients to postoperative intravesical epirubicin or no treatment groups, and found benefit in those patients whose EORTC risk score was 0–2, but no benefit in those with risk scores of three or more [7]. Despite this, a single postoperative instillation of mitomycin has been adopted as standard practice in Europe. Further data confirm the benefit of repeated instillations, and a single instillation may be insufficient for patients with multifocal disease. These tumors, which are classified as intermediate risks for recurrence, can be treated with a prolonged 6-week course of mitomycin at a dose of 40 mg in 40 ml sterile water. Such treatment is safe and effective in reducing the risk of recurrence in the short term, but the efficacy is only marginal in the long term [8]. Despite repeated dosing, prolonged instillation of mitomycin does not appear to reduce the risk of tumor progression. A meta-analysis of nine clinical trials

TABLE 1.3. Toxicity of intravesical Bacillus Calmette-Guerin (BCG) and mitomycin C (adapted from 1999 American Urological Association guidelines).

Toxicity	Mitomycin	BCG
Local		
Frequency/nocturia	42% (26–59%)	63% (48–76%)
Dysuria	35% (30–41%)	75% (64–84%)
Urgency	18% (12–26%)	Too varied
Pain/cramps	10% (6–14%)	12% (7–18%)
Hematuria	16% (7–28%)	29% (22–36%)
Incontinence	1% (0.4–4%)	4% (3–6%)
Bladder contracture	5% (2–11%)	3% (2–5%)
Systemic		
Flu-like illness	20% (4–48%)	24% (18–31%)
Fever/chills	3% (1–7%)	27% (22–32%)
Arthalgia	9% (0.1–47%)	5% (1–13%)
Myelosuppression	2% (0.3–7%)	1% (0.1–4%)
Nausea/vomiting	9% (1–26%)	9% (6–14%)
Skin rash	13% (8–19%)	6% (3–10%)
Other	3% (0.5–8%)	23% (19–27%)
Infectious		
Bacterial cystitis	20% (17–23%)	20% (13–8%)
Epididymitis/prostatitis/urethritis	4% (2–9%)	5% (4–8%)
Pneumonia	0.2% (0–2%)	1% (0.2–3%)
Systemic	NR	4% (2–5%)
Treatment continuation rates		
Incomplete	9% (2–14%)	8% (5–10%)
Interruption	11% (8–16%)	7% (5–11%)

compared its efficacy on progression with that of the immunotherapy agent, Bacillus Calmette-Guerin (BCG). With a median follow-up of 26 months, 7.7% of the patients in the BCG group and 9.4% of the patients in the mitomycin group developed tumor progression [9]. The main side effects of mitomycin are described in Table 1.3.

Other Intravesical Chemotherapy Agents

Alternative agents have been tested and can be used when mitomycin is contraindicated and as second-line therapy. One of the earliest intravesical therapies for urothelial carcinoma was triethylene thiophosphoramide, or thiotepa, which produces a reduction in the recurrence of bladder tumors by 25%, when compared with recurrence after transurethral resection alone [10]. It is used infrequently, however, as a result of potential bone marrow suppression due to systemic absorption attributed to its low molecular weight. Another seldom-used intravesical agent is doxorubicin, an antitumor antibiotic, which inhibits DNA synthesis through intercalation. It reduces tumor recurrence by up to 40% and carries fewer adverse effects than thiotepa, due to higher molecular weight [11]. Epirubicin is a synthetic modification of doxorubicin, which some patients will not tolerate due to adverse effects, but all grades of NMIBC experience a reduction in recurrence by up to 50%.

Other less commonly used intravesical chemotherapeutic agents which have been described as second-line treatments in selected patients include mitoxantrone, offering the benefit of similar efficacy but with less instillations, and valrubicin.

Optimizing Intravesical Mitomycin

Methods to optimize mitomycin have been reported and can be adopted. Eliminating residual urine volume, overnight fasting, using sodium bicarbonate to reduce drug degradation, and increasing concentration to 40 mg in 20 ml have all been used [12]. Recently, a randomized trial reported that increased drug temperature through the use of local microwave therapy is effective as a combination therapy. In a randomized trial, hyperthermia plus mitomycin reduced the recurrence of NMIBC from 57.5 to 17.1% [13]. Other studies seem to confirm the benefit of microwave hyperthermia with even higher doses of mitomycin (40–80 mg) for 6–8 weeks in high-grade bladder cancer [14,15]. Bladder wall hyperthermia of 42–43°C can be achieved with a catheter containing internal thermocouples to monitor the temperature. Long-term follow-up will clearly help to determine the role of this new technology.

Electromotive drug administration (EMDA) enhances penetration of drugs through the use of an electrical gradient between the bladder wall and its contents. Di Stasi et al. [16]

compared mitomycin only, mitomycin with EMDA, and BCG in 108 high-risk patients and obtained complete responses in 31, 58, and 64%, respectively, after 6 months follow-up. The side effects of mitomycin with EMDA were more than with mitomycin alone, but less than those with BCG. Again, this is a therapy that is not currently a mainstream one, but may find its place in the treatment algorithm in the future.

Intravesical Bacillus Calmette-Guerin (BCG) Immunotherapy

BCG is an attenuated *Mycobacterium bovis*, which exhibits an antitumor activity. The original protocol described by Morales et al. included a percutaneous dose that allowed for the skin reaction to be monitored as an indicator of bladder response. The effects noted by weeks 4–5 were not further enhanced by more BCG administration, and on this basis, the 6-week course was established. The percutaneous dose was discontinued after subsequent success using intravesical therapy alone [17].

Only intravesical BCG has been shown to reduce the risk of stage progression in NMIBC. BCG induces a local immune response when bound by fibronectin within the bladder wall. As a result, a T-cell-mediated immune reaction ensues following the activation of dendritic cells and Th1-type cytokines (interferon-γ and IL-2), which mediate cytotoxic natural killer cell and direct cytoxicity. The initial response rate is up to 80%, although only around 50% of the patients experience a durable response over 4 years, and when followed for 10 years, this figure falls to 30%. Herr et al. found progression in 19% of those who responded to BCG at 5 years, but 95% in nonresponders [18].

Sylvester et al. performed a meta-analysis of the published results of randomized clinical trials by comparing the transurethral resection plus intravesical BCG vs. resection alone or resection plus another treatment other than BCG [19]. The meta-analysis included 24 trials with progression information on 4,863 patients. Based on a median follow-up of 2.5 years and a maximum of 15 years, 9.8% of the patients on BCG exhibited progression when compared with 13.8% patients in the control groups, equivalent to a reduction of 27% in the odds of progression on BCG. The number of cases that progressed was low (6.4% of 2,880 patients with papillary tumors and 13.9% of 403 patients with CIS) and the data must be interpreted with some caution; however, only patients receiving maintenance BCG benefited. Although there was no significant difference in the treatment effect on either overall survival or death due to bladder cancer, the authors concluded that BCG is the agent of choice for patients with intermediate and high-risk papillary tumors and those with CIS.

In a randomized trial of 86 patients with high-risk NMIBC, Herr [20] showed a longer interval to progression for BCG-treated patients when compared with the controls, and demonstrated that the rate of progressing to cystectomy was lower for CIS patients treated with BCG (11% for BCG treated group when compared with 55% for controls). A key point to be stressed, however, is that with a longer-term follow-up of 10–15 years, only 27% of the patients remained alive with bladder preserved. Clearly, BCG can delay the progression of NMIBC, but the option of primary cystectomy must be considered, especially in young patients with aggressive disease. If after an induction course of six instillations, there has been no response, a second induction may achieve a response in 25% of the patients with high-grade papillary disease and 30% of the patients with CIS. If there is no response to the second induction, then the clinical outcome is not favorable, and further BCG is not recommended [21].

The Southwest Oncology Group (SWOG) first reported the effect of maintenance therapy in a randomized trial. A total of 550 patients were randomized to receive BCG maintenance therapy or no BCG maintenance therapy. The maintenance regimen consisted of intravesical and percutaneous BCG each week for 3 weeks, given at 3, 6, 12, 18, 24, 30, and 36 months. The median recurrence-free survival was 35.7 months in the non-maintenance and 76.8 months in the maintenance arm. The overall 5-year survival was 78% in the non-maintenance arm, when compared with 83% in the maintenance arm. The authors concluded that maintenance BCG was more effective than induction therapy alone. This view is now widely accepted and most patients will begin their BCG therapy with a plan to provide a maintenance regimen. Further studies to determine the optimal duration of maintenance have been completed by the EORTC and the answer will become clear in the next 5 years. The main side effects of BCG therapy are described in Table 1.3.

Accurate Detection and Clearance of NMIBC

Recently, there has been renewed interest in the use of photo-dynamic therapy and detection in bladder cancer. Photosensitive compounds are instilled into the bladder, which are preferentially taken up by the tumor cells. The bladder is then illuminated with blue ultraviolet light at 450 nm, which is absorbed and emitted at a longer wavelength of 650 nm, by tumor which fluoresces red under the blue light. The currently used photosensitizer is hexyl 5-aminolevulinic acid. Filbeck [22] demonstrated in a randomized controlled trial that recurrence after TURBT at 1 year could be reduced from 26% to 10.5% and it is estimated that 20–30% more tumors are detected using this technology. Whether this translates into a reduction in disease progression or improved long-term survival is still unclear, but there may be a role for this technique in cases of unexplained positive cytology. 5-amino-levulinic acid has been used in therapy in phase I trials, which showed promising early results.

Clinical Application of Medical Therapies

A simplified clinical management flowchart describing when adjuvant chemotherapy and immunotherapy should be administered is presented in Fig. 1.1, and is based on the consensus guidelines developed by the European Association of Urology [23]. It is standard practice to administer one single instillation of intravesical chemotherapy following TURBT; and this should ideally be delivered within 6 h of surgery. All available intravesical chemotherapeutic agents are similarly effective,

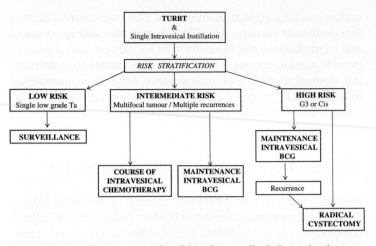

FIGURE 1.1.   Management algorithm for medical therapies in non-muscle invasive bladder cancer (NMIBC).

but differ in their associated adverse effects. Mitomycin is the most commonly used agent in this setting in the UK.

For multiple recurrences or multifocal disease, a course of intravesical chemotherapy or BCG induction plus maintenance may be considered. The optimal chemotherapeutic instillation schedule remains unknown. Generally, a course of six instillations of chemotherapy are used in this setting.

For those with high-grade disease or CIS, BCG induction followed by maintenance therapy using the SWOG maintenance schedule is initiated following TURBT. BCG treatment should be started at least 2 weeks after TURBT, to reduce the risk of systemic complications. BCG is not indicated for muscle invasive disease, as for this disease, radical treatment is advised. Early "second-look" re-resection of the tumor base to confirm staging in the case of T1G3 disease, is performed prior to considering BCG treatment.

The SWOG maintenance schedule consists of induction (6-weekly instillations of BCG) followed by 3-weekly instillations at 3 and 6 months, and then every 6 months for 3 years. The optimal duration of maintenance therapy is not clear, but all guidelines recommend at least 1 year of therapy.

Patients who relapse following BCG maintenance (either recurrence or progression) should strongly consider radical treatment options.

Experimental therapies which may be considered for nonindex patients in trial settings include thermochemotherapy and EMDA.

Key Points

1. A single postoperative instillation of chemotherapeutic agent reduces the risk of recurrence following TURBT by 39%.
2. Intravesical chemotherapy (usually mitomycin) should be given within 6 h where possible.
3. Following TURBT, patients should be assigned to a risk group and given adjuvant intravesical treatment where appropriate.
4. Intravesical chemotherapy does not prevent progression, but maintenance BCG reduces the risk of progression of high-risk NMIBC by 27%.
5. Failure of intravesical BCG treatment warrants consideration of radical treatment options.

References

1. Donat SM (2003) Evaluation and follow-up strategies for superficial bladder cancer. Urol Clin North Am 30(4):765–766
2. Sylvester RJ, van der Meijden AP, Oosterlinck W, Witjes JA, Bouffioux C, Denis L, Newling DW, Kurth K (2006) Predicting recurrence and progression in individual patients with stage Ta T1 bladder cancer using EORTC risk tables: a combined analysis of 2596 patients from seven EORTC trials. Eur Urol 49(3):466–475; discussion 475–477
3. Veerakumarasivam A, Scott HE, Chin SF, Warren A, Wallard MJ, Grimmer D, Ichimura K, Caldas C, Collins VP, Neal DE, Kelly JD (2008) High-resolution array-based comparative genomic hybridization of bladder cancers identifies mouse double minute 4 (MDM4) as an amplification target exclusive of MDM2 and TP53. Clin Cancer Res 14(9):2527–2534

4. Gasion JP, Cruz JF (2006) Improving efficacy of intravesical chemotherapy. Eur Urol 50(2):225–234

5. Tolley DA, Hargreave TB, Smith PH, Williams JL, Grigor KM, Parmar MK, Freedman LS, Uscinska BM (1988) Effect of intravesical mitomycin C on recurrence of newly diagnosed superficial bladder cancer: interim report from the Medical research council subgroup on superficial bladder cancer (urological cancer working party). Br Med J (Clin Res Ed) 296(6639):1759–1761

6. Sylvester RJ, Oosterlinck W, van der Meijden AP (2004) A single immediate postoperative instillation of chemotherapy decreases the risk of recurrence in patients with stage Ta T1 bladder cancer: a meta-analysis of published results of randomized clinical trials. J Urol 171(6 Pt 1):2186–2190; quiz 2435

7. Gudjonsson, S, Adell L, Merdasa F, Olsson R, Larsson B, Davidsson T, Richthoff J, Hagberg G, Grabe M, Bendahl PO, Mansson W, Liedberg F (2009) Should all patients with non-muscle-invasive bladder cancer receive early intravesical chemotherapy after transurethral resection? The results of a prospective randomised multicentre study. Eur Urol Apr;55(4):773–80

8. Witjes JA, Hendricksen K (2008) Intravesical pharmacotherapy for non-muscle-invasive bladder cancer: a critical analysis of currently available drugs, treatment schedules, and long-term results. Eur Urol 53(1):45–52

9. Bohle A, Bock PR (2004) Intravesical Bacille Calmette-Guerin versus mitomycin C in superficial bladder cancer: formal meta-analysis of comparative studies on tumor progression. Urology 63(4): 682–686; discussion 686–687

10. Kurth K, Tunn U, Ay R, Schroder FH, Pavone-Macaluso M, Debruyne F, ten Kate F, de Pauw M, Sylvester R (1997) Adjuvant chemotherapy for superficial transitional cell bladder carcinoma: long-term results of a European organization for research and treatment of cancer randomized trial comparing doxorubicin, ethoglucid and transurethral resection alone. J Urol 158(2):378–384

11. Brassell SA, Kamat AM (2006) Contemporary intravesical treatment options for urothelial carcinoma of the bladder. J Natl Compr Canc Netw 4(10):1027–1036

12. Au JL, Badalament RA, Wientjes MG, Young DC, Warner JA, Venema PL, Pollifrone DL, Harbrecht JD, Chin JL, Lerner SP, Miles BJ (2001) Methods to improve efficacy of intravesical mitomycin C: results of a randomized phase III trial. J Natl Cancer Inst 93(8):597–604

13. Colombo R, Da Pozzo LF, Salonia A, Rigatti P, Leib Z, Baniel J, Caldarera E, Pavone-Macaluso M (2003) Multicentric study comparing intravesical chemotherapy alone and with local microwave hyperthermia for prophylaxis of recurrence of superficial transitional cell carcinoma. J Clin Oncol 21(23):4270–4276

14. Gofrit ON, Shapiro A, Pode D, Sidi A, Nativ O, Leib Z, Witjes JA, van der Heijden AG, Naspro R, Colombo R (2004) Combined local bladder hyperthermia and intravesical chemotherapy for the treatment of high-grade superficial bladder cancer. Urology 63(3):466–471

15. van der Heijden AG, Kiemeney LA, Gofrit ON, Nativ O, Sidi A, Leib Z, Colombo R, Naspro R, Pavone M, Baniel J, Hasner F, Witjes JA (2004) Preliminary European results of local microwave hyperthermia and chemotherapy treatment in intermediate or high risk superficial transitional cell carcinoma of the bladder. Eur Urol 46(1):65–71; discussion 71–72

16. Di Stasi SM, Giannantoni A, Stephen RL, Capelli G, Navarra P, Massoud R, Vespasiani G (2003) Intravesical electromotive mitomycin C versus passive transport mitomycin C for high risk superficial bladder cancer: a prospective randomized study. J Urol 170(3):777–782

17. Morales A, Eidinger D, Bruce AW (1976) Intracavitary Bacillus Calmette-Guerin in the treatment of superficial bladder tumors. J Urol 116(2):180–183

18. Herr HW, Badalament RA, Amato DA, Laudone VP, Fair WR, Whitmore WF Jr (1989) Superficial bladder cancer treated with Bacillus Calmette-Guerin: a multivariate analysis of factors affecting tumor progression. J Urol 141(1):22–29

19. Sylvester RJ, van der MA, Lamm DL (2002) Intravesical bacillus Calmette-Guerin reduces the risk of progression in patients with superficial bladder cancer: a meta-analysis of the published results of randomized clinical trials. J Urol 168(5):1964–1970

20. Herr HW, Laudone VP, Badalament RA, Oettgen HF, Sogani PC, Freedman BD, Melamed MR, Whitmore WF Jr (1988) Bacillus Calmette-Guerin therapy alters the progression of superficial bladder cancer. J Clin Oncol 6(9):1450–1455

21. Nadler RB, Catalona WJ, Hudson MA, Ratliff TL (1994) Durability of the tumor-free response for intravesical Bacillus Calmette-Guerin therapy. J Urol 152(2 Pt 1):367–373

22. Filbeck T, Pichlmeier U, Knuechel R, Wieland WF, Roessler W (2002) Clinically relevant improvement of recurrence-free

survival with 5-aminolevulinic acid induced fluorescence diagnosis in patients with superficial bladder tumors. J Urol 168(1):67–71

23. Babjuk M, Oosterlinck W, Sylvester R, Kaasinen E, Bohle A, Palou-Redorta J (2008) EAU guidelines on non-muscle-invasive urothelial carcinoma of the bladder. Eur Urol 54(2):303–314

Chapter 2
Renal Cell Cancer

Bryan Y. Wong and Wolfram E. Samlowski

Introduction

Cancers of the kidney account for 3–4% of new adult malignancies in the United States and Europe. In 2008, it is estimated that there will be over 208,000 new cases diagnosed worldwide, leading to more than 102,000 deaths. At presentation, 30% of patients have metastatic disease, and 50% of patients with localized disease will subsequently develop metastases. Metastatic disease has a poor prognosis with a 5-year survival of <10% [1]. Metastatic cancer remains a therapeutic challenge. The failure of standard chemotherapy (renal cancer is resistant to chemotherapy agents ascribed to high expression levels of the multidrug resistance, MDR1, gene), and the modest success of immunotherapy has necessitated the requirement for other strategies to manage the disease.

Molecular Pathogenesis of Renal Cancer

Hereditary risk factors have been identified, and molecular genetic studies have identified the responsible genetic mutations. These studies have been informative with regard to the

W.E. Samlowski (✉)
Section of Renal Cancer and Immunotherapy, Nevada Cancer Institute, One Breakthrough Way, Las Vegas, NV 89135 USA
e-mail: wsamlowski@nvcancer.org

I.S. Shergill et al. (eds.), *Medical Therapy in Urology*,
DOI 10.1007/978-1-84882-704-2_2,
© Springer-Verlag London Limited 2010

pathogenesis of nonfamilial renal cancer. The same genetic pathways that are affected in rare patients with familial cancer syndromes are frequently affected by somatic mutations or inactivation in sporadic cancer. Familial studies of patients with Von Hippel-Lindau (VHL) syndrome (hemangioblastomas, pheochromocytomas, renal and hepatic cysts, clear cell renal cancer) identified mutations in a novel gene termed VHL. The protein encoded by VHL mediates the rapid degradation of a family of hypoxia-induced transcription factors (HIF) under normoxic conditions. Mutations in VHL lead to an over-accumulation of HIF-1α and HIF-2α, which mediate signals leading to tumor angiogenesis (e.g., increases in vascular endothelial growth factor (VEGF); platelet derived growth factor, PDGF) and overexpression of other cell proteins (e.g., erythropoeitin, glucose transporter-1, CA-IX). Inactivation of the VHL pathway was subsequently identified in over 70% of sporadic renal clear cell tumors. An alternative pathway of renal carcinogenesis involves activation of the mammalian target of rapamycin (mTOR). This pathway links the extracellular signals (e.g., via insulin or insulin-like growth factors) with cell proliferation and growth. mTOR activity is modulated by other oncogenes, such as phosphoinoside (PI)-3-kinase, AKT, PTEN, and the tuberous sclerosis complex (TSC). These observations provided the rationale for the development of small-molecule inhibitors of these pathways.

Prognostic Factors

The clinical stage remains the single most important predictor of survival and outcome in renal cancer (Table. 2.1 – TNM classification). However, in metastatic disease, a number of clinical features have been identified as powerful independent variables predicting the outcome. Patients are classified as good, intermediate, and poor risk, depending upon whether they possess zero, one, or two or more of the following risk factors: Karnofsky performance status ≤ 80%, anemia, elevated serum calcium, absence of prior nephrec-

TABLE 2.1   Contemporary TNM staging of renal carcinoma†

T	Primary tumor stage
Tx	Tumor extent cannot be assessed
T0	No evidence of primary tumor
T1	
T1a	Tumor ≤4 cm, confined within renal capsule
T1b	Tumor 4-7 cm, confined within renal capsule
T2	Tumor ≥7 cm, confined within renal capsule
T3	
T3a	Tumor directly invades adrenal gland or peri-nephric fat but not beyond Gerota's fascia
T3b	Tumor extends into the renal vein or vena cava (below diaphragm)
T3c	Tumor extends into vena cava (above diaphragm) or has grown into wall of vena cava
T4	Tumor extends beyond Gerota's fascia
N	**Nodal involvement**
NX	Regional lymph nodes cannot be assessed
N0	No regional lymph node metastasis
N1	Metastasis in a single regional lymph node
N2	Metastasis in more than one regional lymph node
M	**Metastases**
M0	Distant metastases absent
M1	Distant metastases present

Stage Groupings	TNM	Estimated 5 year survival
Stage I	T1a-T1b, N0, M0	96%
Stage II	T2, N0, M0	82%
Stage III	T3a-T3c and/or N1, M0	64%
Stage IV	T4, N0 or N1, M0	
	Any T, N2, M0	
	Any T, Any N and M1	23%*

†Derived from American Joint Committee on Cancer TNM staging system 2002.
*5-year survival in stage IV disease is currently a moving target, due to advent of a large number of active agents

tomy, and elevated lactate dehydrogenase [2]. Multiorgan involvement is also associated with decreased survival. Survival is approximately 20, 10, and 4 months in patients with 0, 1, or ≥2 risk factors.

Medical Therapies in Renal Cancer

The Immunotherapy Era (1984–2004)

Interferon-α (IFNα)

IFNα is a cytokine that activates natural killer (NK) cells, enhances antigen expression by cancer cells, and is antiproliferative in vitro. Clinical studies suggest an overall response rate of approximately 10–20% following treatment of renal cancer with subcutaneous or intravenous IFNα for 3–5 days per week. Onset of response is slow, median response duration is approximately 6 months, and complete responses are rare. IFNα administration results in substantial chronic toxicity, including "flu-like" symptoms, fatigue, nausea, diarrhea, rash, pruritus, and depression [3].

Interleukin-2 (IL-2)

The cytokine IL-2 was discovered on account of its ability to strongly induce lymphocyte cytotoxicity in vitro. Initial studies demonstrated that high-dose intravenous IL-2 in combination with IL-2-activated lymphocytes (lymphokine-activated killer or LAK cells) produced rare but dramatic complete and partial responses in patients with metastatic renal cancer and melanoma [4]. Subsequent studies showed that most of the antitumor activity was derived from IL-2. Low subcutaneous doses of IL-2 have similar activity to IFNα and megesterol acetate [3]. Current estimates suggest that the objective response rate to high-dose IL-2 is 15–20%, with a durable complete response rate of 5–7%. Many of the complete responders remain in long-term durable remissions (decades). The major limitation of high-dose IL-2 treatment is severe toxicity in virtually every organ system. This includes severe hypotension, vascular leak syndrome, neuropsychiatric toxicity, and many others. Therefore, close clinical monitoring in an intensive care unit setting is required. The optimal patients for IL-2 treatment have excellent performance status (without cardiac or pulmonary co-morbidity) and clear cell tumors. Patients whose tumors overexpress carbonic anhydrase IX (CA-IX) may also have an increased response probability.

Targeted Therapies in Renal Cell Carcinoma (2004 to Present)

Sorafenib

Sorafenib (Nexavar®) is an oral ATP-mimetic multikinase inhibitor. Targets include c-RAF, b-RAF, as well as the VEGF receptor (VEGFR)-2 and -3, platelet derived growth factor receptor (PDGFR) beta, FLT3, cKIT, and fibroblast growth factor receptor (FGFR)-1 tyrosine kinases. This agent unexpectedly demonstrated activity against renal cancer and hepatoma. A randomized phase III study was performed, comparing sorafenib against placebo in 903 patients after initial cytokine failure [5]. The majority were low- and intermediate-risk patients with clear cell histology. Although sorafenib produced a low objective response rate (10%), prolongation of median progression-free survival (~6 months vs. 3 months) was found. Even though there was a trend toward greater median overall survival, this did not reach statistical significance, due to crossover of patients on the placebo arm to active agents. Therapy was well-tolerated, with mild diarrhea, hand–foot skin reactions, hypertension, and hair graying as side effects. These findings led to regulatory approval. Subsequently, a phase II trial in previously untreated metastatic renal cancer did not show superiority of sorafenib over IFNα.

Sunitinib

Sunitinib is another oral multikinase inhibitor. This agent inhibits VEGFR-1, 2 and 3, PDGFR-alpha and beta, FGFR-1, c-KIT, and FLT3. A pair of phase II studies in patients with previously treated metastatic RCC demonstrated objective response rates of 34 and 40%, with progression-free survivals of more than 8 months. In addition, nearly 30% of the patients, who did not have objective responses, demonstrated prolonged disease stability. The toxicity profile for sunitinib included stomatitis, nausea and vomiting, diarrhea, hypertension, hand–foot skin reaction, neutropenia, anemia, thrombocytopenia, and amylase elevations. Additional toxicities include frequent hypothyroidism and, rarely, decreased myocardial ejection fraction. The latter infrequently results in overt congestive heart failure and is usually reversible with drug discontinuation. A large randomized phase III study was performed, randomizing good and intermediate risk, previously untreated patients, to receive either sunitinib or IFNα [6]. Sunitinib demonstrated superior activity (response rate 39% vs. 8%) and improved progression-free survival (11 vs. 5 months). Overall survival analysis favored sunitinib (26.4 vs. 21.8 months), and achieved borderline statistical significance ($p = 0.051$). Survival results were again confounded by crossover from IFNα to sunitinib and other active agents. Based on these results, sunitinib is currently the most frequent first-line therapy for metastatic renal cancer in the United States.

Bevacizumab

It is believed that for tumor growth and progression to occur, there is a necessity for concomitant growth of tumor neovasculature (angiogenesis). Bevacizumab, a humanized monoclonal antibody was developed to target VEGF. This molecule has demonstrated significant antitumor activity across a number of malignancies, including colorectal cancer, nonsmall cell lung cancer, breast cancer, and more recently, glioblastoma multiforme. In addition, early studies demonstrated its activity in renal cancer. A randomized phase II study in patients with metastatic RCC who had failed prior IL-2 treatment demonstrated a 10% partial response rate at the highest dose of bevacizumab [7]. This was associated with a modestly increased time to progression (4.8 vs. 2 months with placebo). In two subsequent phase III trials (AVOREN and CALGB 90206), previously untreated patients were randomized to receive low doses of IFNα in combination with bevacizumab or placebo [8]. The bevacizumab arms of both the trials proved superior, with objective response rates of 21 and 31%. Progression-free survival was also significantly improved over IFNα alone (approximately 10 months). Unfortunately, neither of the trials contained a bevacizumab alone arm, to assess the importance of this agent. These results suggest that the activity of the bevacizumab/IFNα combination approaches that of single agent activity of sunitinib. This combination has substantial toxicity, mostly related to IFNα. Unique toxicities of bevacizumab include hypertension and proteinuria (sometimes leading to nephrotic syndrome). Rare, but serious toxicities include risk of bleeding at tumor sites and thromboses.

Temsirolimus

The mTOR pathway is modulated by the oncogenes PI-3-kinase, AKT, PTEN, and TSC, which are all believed to be relevant to renal cancer growth. Recent studies have also shown that mTOR may also modulate the HIF pathway (and tumor angiogenesis). Analogs of the immunosuppressive agent rapamycin, such as temsirolimus, were found to block mTOR function. Temsirolimus was subsequently tested in a randomized phase II study in renal cancer. This study did not identify a maximum tolerated dose and appeared to show the greatest benefit in intermediate- and poor-risk renal cancer patients. This led to a large phase III study of 626 patients with untreated, metastatic, poor-prognosis renal cancer [9]. Patients were randomized to receive temsirolimus, IFNα, or both. Of note, this study included 20% nonclear cell histology patients. Response rates were not statistically different between the arms; however, single-agent temsirolimus demonstrated significantly prolonged overall survival (10.9 months) and progression-free survival (5.5 months). Single-agent temsirolimus was well tolerated, and was associated with skin rash, mucositis, asthenia (loss of energy and appetite), nausea, hyperglycemia, hypertriglyceridemia, hypophosphatemia, and anemia. Rare toxicities include thromboses and interstitial pneumonitis.

Everolimus

The success of temsirolimus led to the development and testing of additional mTOR inhibitors. Everolimus is one such oral analog. In a recent phase III study in renal cancer, 410 patients who had failed at least one kinase inhibitor were randomized in a 2:1 fashion to everolimus vs. placebo [10]. The results of this trial showed an improved progression-free survival when compared with the results with placebo (4.0 vs. 1.9 months). This agent is therefore approved for use in patients with prior VEGFR inhibitor failure.

Cytotoxic Chemotherapy

Historically, RCC has been felt to be resistant to conventional cytotoxic chemotherapy (e.g., to vinblastine) or hormonal agents (megesterol acetate) due to high expression of multidrug transport proteins. Recent data suggest modest responses to gemcitabine-based therapy in combination with 5-flurouracil, capecitibine, or doxorubicin, particularly in patients with non-clear cell tumors.

Cytoreductive Nephrectomy

Cytoreductive nephrectomy may be indicated for palliation, to prevent or decrease local and systemic symptoms in patients presenting with metastatic disease at the time of diagnosis of a renal primary. In the era of cytokine therapy, a survival benefit of cytoreductive nephrectomy followed by IFNα treatment was demonstrated in two randomized clinical trials, independent of patient performance status, the site of metastases, and the presence of measurable disease [11,12]. The EORTC study showed that median survival with IFNα and nephrectomy (18 months) was significantly better than IFNα alone (11 months) [11]. The SWOG also reported that nephrectomy followed by interferon therapy resulted in significantly longer median survival among patients with metastatic renal-cell cancer than interferon therapy alone (11 vs. 8 months) [12]. Subsequently, a combined analysis of the SWOG and EORTC trials was published in 2004 [13]. In this combined report, data were available on 331 patients, randomized to nephrectomy followed by IFNα, as opposed to IFNα alone and the median survival was 13.6 vs. 7.8 months, respectively. This difference represented a 31% decrease in the risk of death ($p = 0.002$). The role of cytoreductive nephrectomy or presurgical cytoreductive therapy in the "targeted therapy era" are currently being evaluated in ongoing clinical trials.

Adjuvant Therapy

Following surgery, it is possible to identify patients who have a high risk for recurrence or metastases, based on the stage and tumor characteristics. The UCLA Integrated Staging System (UISS) incorporates TNM staging with performance status and histologic grade to divide patients into five prognostic categories [14]. The role of postoperative adjuvant therapy has been investigated. Agents such IFNα and IL-2 have not produced a survival benefit. Studies investigating the newer "targeted therapy" in the adjuvant setting are currently ongoing. Apart from clinical trials, there is currently no evidence-based rationale for adjuvant therapy in locally advanced renal cancer.

Current Treatment Strategies and Ongoing Investigations

Current treatment strategies may include quite a number of active agents (Table 2.2). A currently employed schema for first- and second-line treatment of metastatic renal cancer has been provided (Figs. 2.1 and 2.2). Numerous additional agents are currently being evaluated in clinical trials in metastatic renal cancer [15,16]. These include active second generation VEGFR kinase inhibitors, such as axitinib and pazopanib, which may have enhanced response rates and a different spectrum of toxicity. Additional mTOR inhibitors and agents that target the PI-3-kinase, AKT, cMET, and other targets are also being tested against renal cancer. Mechanisms of resistance to VEGFR and mTOR pathway inhibitors are not yet known. Cross-resistance does not appear to be absolute. Thus, it may be possible to utilize multiple kinase inhibitors in succession [15,16]. While combinations of multiple VEGF pathway

TABLE 2.2. Medical therapies for metastatic renal cancer.

Name	Mode of action	Dose	Main side effects	Interactions/contraindications
Interleukin-2 (IL-2)	Cytokine, immune modulation	600,000 IU/kg IV TDS over 15 min– days 1–5 and 14–18, on a 12 week cycle	Hypotension, vascular leak syndrome, edema, dyspnea, arrhythmia, renal dysfunction, neurotoxicity, nausea/vomiting, infection, rash, lethargy	Hypersensitivity to IL-2/components, cardiac, pulmonary impairment; renal, hepatic, CNS impairment, organ allograft, autoimmune disorders, seizures, bowel ischemia, perforation; caution with corticosteroids
Sorafenib	Small molecule, inhibits VEGFR, PDGFR, FLT3, cKIT, FGFR, C-RAF, B-RAF (anti-angiogenesis)	400 mg PO BD	Hypertension, skin rash, hand–foot skin reaction, diarrhea, fatigue, nausea, acne, dry mouth	Hypersensitivity; caution in pts with hypertension, history of hemorrhage, cardiovascular disease, recent surgery; caution in patients on drugs affecting liver enzymes
Sunitinib	Small molecule, inhibits VEGFR, PDGFR, FLT3, cKIT, FGFR, SRC, IGFR (antiangiogenesis)	50 mg PO QDS for 28 days, then 14 days off	Hypertension, skin rash, diarrhea, nausea/vomiting, cytopenias	Hypersensitivity; caution in pts with cardiovascular disease, hypertension, hemorrhagic events, recent surgery; cardiac arrhythmia
Temsirolimus	mTOR inhibitor	25 mg iv weekly	Fatigue, nausea, skin rash, stomatitis, hyperglycemia, hyperlipidemia, edema, nausea, cytopenias, liver/renal dysfunction	Hypersensitivity; caution in pts with bowel perforation, hemorrhage, hyperglycemia, hyperlipidemia, renal dysfunction

	Mechanism	Dose	Side effects	Cautions
Interferon-alpha (IFNα)	Cytokine, immune modulation	5–10 million units sc qd 6–18 million units sc three times weekly	Flu-like symptoms, fevers, chills, myalgias, fatigue, depression, cytopenias, abnormal liver function studies, nausea/vomiting, injection site reactions	Hypersensitivity to IFN-A/components, autoimmune disorders, hepatitis; caution in pts with cardiovascular and pulmonary disease, diabetes, seizures coagulopathy, myelosuppression, mood disturbance
Bevacizumab	monoclonal antibody against VEGF (antiangiogenesis)	10 mg/kg IV q2 weeks	Hypertension, proteinuria, GI or tumor bleeding, thromboembolic disease, malaise	Caution in pts with recent surgery, history hemorrhage, thromboembolic disease, cardiovascular disease, proteinuria
Axitinib	Small molecule, inhibits VEGFR, PDGFR	5 mg p.o. bd	Hypertension, fatigue, stomatitis, skin rash	Caution in pts with recent surgery, history hemorrhage, thromboembolic disease, cardiovascular disease
Pazopanib	Small molecule, inhibits VEGFR, PDGFR, KIT (antiangiogenesis)	800 mg p.o. qd	Fatigue, diarrhea, rash, abnormal liver function studies, nausea	Caution in pts with recent surgery, history hemorrhage, thromboembolic disease, cardiovascular disease
Everolimus	mTOR inhibitor	10 mg p.o. qd	Skin rash, fatigue, hyperglycemia, hyperlipidemia	Caution in pts with hyperlipidemia, hyperglycemia

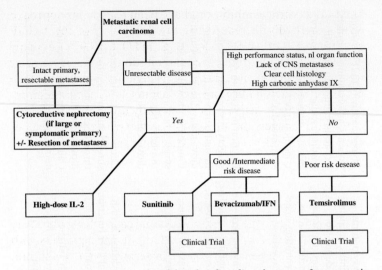

FIGURE 2.1.   Treatment algorithm for *first-line* therapy of metastatic renal cancer.

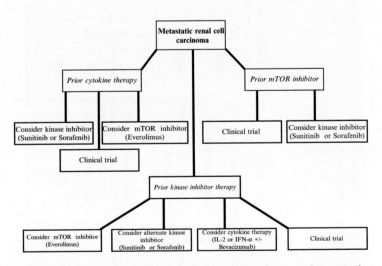

FIGURE 2.2.   Treatment algorithm for *second-line* therapy of metastatic renal cancer.

inhibitors (vertical inhibition) have been tested, this approach yields markedly increased toxicity. Inhibition of the VEGF pathway plus other pathways (e.g., mTOR, EGFR) appears to be more tolerable (horizontal inhibition). It is not yet clear whether combination therapy yields benefits superior to those from the sequential use of single agents. With the large number of potentially active agents currently under trial, it is likely that the management strategies for metastatic renal cancer may be modified, even in the immediate future [15,16].

Key Points

1. Treatment options for advanced renal cancer have markedly improved over recent years, and importantly, patients with metastatic cancer should be characterized as good, intermediate, or poor risk.
2. Good- and intermediate-risk patients should be initially treated with sunitinib or bevacizumab plus IFNα. Selected high-performance status patients with clear cell tumors can be considered for high-dose IL-2.
3. Second-line therapy after progression could include sorafenib, everolimus, or a different VEGF pathway inhibitor.
4. Poor-risk patients, especially those with nonclear cell histology, should initially be considered for treatment with temsirolimus.
5. Clinical trials are strongly recommended for patients failing mTOR inhibitors, those with nonclear cell histology, or after second-line treatment failure.

References

1. Escudier B, Eisen T, Stadler WM et al (2007) Sorafenib in advanced clear-cell renal-cell carcinoma. N Engl J Med 356:125–134
2. Escudier B, Pluzanska A, Koralewski P et al (2007) Bevacizumab plus interferon alfa-2a for treatment of metastatic renal cell carcinoma: a randomised, double-blind phase III trial. Lancet 370:2103–2111

3. Flanigan RC, Salmon SE, Blumenstein BA, Bearman SI, Roy V, McGrath PC, Caton JR Jr, Munshi N, Crawford ED (2001) Nephrectomy followed by interferon alfa-2b compared with interferon alfa-2b alone for metastatic renal cell cancer. N Engl J Med 345(23):1655–1659

4. Flanigan RC, Mickisch G, Sylvester R et al (2004) Cytoreductive nephrectomy in patients with metastatic renal cancer: a combined analysis. J Urol 171:1071–1076

5. Hudes G, Carducci M, Tomczak P et al (2007) Temsirolimus, interferon alfa, or both for advanced renal-cell carcinoma. N Engl J Med 356:2271–2281

6. Lotze MT, Chang AE, Seipp CA et al (1986) High-dose recombinant interleukin 2 in the treatment of patients with disseminated cancer. Responses, treatment-related morbidity, and histologic findings. JAMA 256:3117–3124

7. Mickisch GH, Garin A, van Poppel H, de Prijck L, Sylvester R (2001) European Organisation for Research and Treatment of Cancer (EORTC) Genitourinary Group. Radical nephrectomy plus interferon-alfa-based immunotherapy compared with interferon-alfa alone in metastatic renal-cell carcinoma: a randomised trial. Lancet 358(9286):966–970

8. Motzer RJ, Bander NH, Nanus DM (1996) Renal cell carcinoma. N Engl J Med 335:865–875

9. Motzer RJ, Mazumdar M, Bacik J et al (1999) Survival and prognostic stratification of 670 patients with advanced renal cell carcinoma. J Clin Oncol 17:2530–2540

10. Motzer RJ, Hutson TE, Tomczak P et al (2007) Sunitinib versus interferon alfa in metastatic renal-cell carcinoma. N Engl J Med 356:115–124

11. Motzer RJ, Escudier B, Oudard S et al (2008) Efficacy of everolimus in advanced renal cell carcinoma: a double-blind, randomised, placebo-controlled phase III trial. Lancet 372:449–456

12. Negrier S, Perol D, Ravaud A et al (2007) Medroxyprogesterone, interferon alfa-2a, interleukin 2, or combination of both cytokines in patients with metastatic renal carcinoma of intermediate prognosis: results of a randomized controlled trial. Cancer 110:2448–2457

13. Rini BI, Halabi S, Rosenberg JE et al (2008) Bevacizumab plus interferon alfa compared with interferon alfa monotherapy in patients with metastatic renal cell carcinoma: CALGB 90206. J Clin Oncol 26:5422–5428

14. Samlowski WE, Vogelzang NJ (2007) Emerging drugs for the treatment of metastatic renal cancer. Expert Opin Emerg Drugs 12:605–618

15. Samlowski WE, Wong B, Vogelzang NJ (2008) Management of renal cancer in the tyrosine kinase inhibitor era: a view from 3 years on. BJU Int 102:162–165
16. Zisman A, Pantuck AJ, Wieder J et al (2002) Risk group assessment and clinical outcome algorithm to predict the natural history of patients with surgically resected renal cell carcinoma. J Clin Oncol 20:4559–4566

Chapter 3
Prostate Cancer

Ajay Pahuja, Ali Thwaini, Thiaga Nambirajan,
and Patrick F. Keane

Introduction

Prostate cancer (PCa) is a very common disease and one
of the leading causes of cancer-related deaths in men in the
UK. Whilst localized disease is potentially curable, locally
advanced and metastatic disease usually requires the use of
medical treatments, and is associated with higher mortality
rates. Eventually, despite appropriate treatment, a hormone-
independent phenotype usually emerges, leading to a median
overall survival of 23–37 months.

Anatomy and Pathophysiology of the Prostate

The prostate is divided into several zones. McNeal's classification accurately describes the different prostatic zones
according to their embryologic origin, and easily allows an
understanding of the pathophysiology of benign prostate
enlargement and PCa.

The transitional zone comprises 10% of the prostate in a
young man. This will increase in size, pushing the peripheral
zone into what appears to be a prostate capsule at a later stage.
The transitional zone is the site of origin of benign prostate
hyperplasia (BPH). The central zone initially comprises 25%

A. Pahuja (✉)
Department of Urology, Belfast City Hospital, Belfast, UK
e-mail: ajay_pahuja@hotmail.com

I.S. Shergill et al. (eds.), *Medical Therapy in Urology*,
DOI 10.1007/978-1-84882-704-2_3,
© Springer-Verlag London Limited 2010

of the gland and is of Wolffian duct origin (from which also arise the vasa deferentia and seminal vesicles). The peripheral zone initially constitutes 75% of the gland, and is later compressed into a pseudocapsule. It is the site of origin of 75% of PCa. The last zone is the anterior fibromuscular stroma, with little function known so far.

Hormonal Control of the Prostate

Prostate cells are physiologically dependent on androgens to stimulate growth, function, and proliferation. Testosterone, although not tumorigenic, is essential for the growth and perpetuation of tumor cells. The testes are the source of most of the androgens, with only 5–10% derived from adrenal biosynthesis. Testosterone secretion is regulated by the hypothalamic–pituitary–gonadal axis. Figure 3.1 describes the endocrinology of the prostate, and the strategies for androgen deprivation. The hypothalamic luteinizing hormone-releasing hormone (LHRH) stimulates the anterior pituitary gland to release luteinizing hormone (LH) and follicle-stimulating

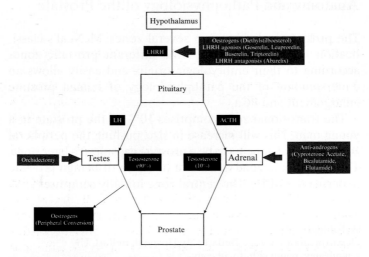

FIGURE 3.1.   Endocrinology of the prostate and sites for medical therapies in prostate cancer (PCa).

hormone (FSH). LH stimulates the Leydig cells of the testes to secrete testosterone. Within the prostate cells, testosterone is converted by the enzyme 5-alpha-reductase into 5-alpha-dihydrotestosterone (DHT), which is an androgenic stimulant approximately ten times more powerful than the parent molecule. Circulating testosterone is peripherally aromatized and converted into estrogens, which, together with the circulating androgens, exert a negative feedback control on the hypothalamic LH secretion.

Androgens influence the development, maturation, and maintenance of the prostate, affecting both the proliferation and differentiation of the luminal epithelium. Ever since the discovery made by Huggins [1] for which he was awarded the Nobel Prize, there has been little doubt that a lifetime of exposure of the prostate to androgens plays an important role in prostate carcinogenesis. Long-term absence of androgen exposure appears to protect the prostate against the development of cancer, but a dose–response relationship between androgen levels and cancer risk has not been established. Hence, the hormonal ablation therapy forms a pivotal role in the management of locally advanced/advanced PCa as shown in Table 3.1.

Medical Therapies in Prostate Cancer

Androgen deprivation therapy (ADT) remains a mainstay of treatment in multiple settings for men with PCa. It was the seminal work of Huggins and Hodges in the early 1940s that formed the cornerstone strategy for the treatment of advanced PCa. They showed that depriving PCa cells of androgens by surgical castration or estrogen treatment could induce programmed cell death (i.e., apoptosis), resulting in major shrinkage of the prostate tumor and its metastases. Bilateral orchiectomy is observed to reduce the testosterone levels very effectively and rapidly. However, surgical castration does have major disadvantages; it is irreversible and can have a profound negative psychological impact on the patient [1].

TABLE 3.1. Medical therapies in prostate cancer (PCa).

Name	Mode of action	Dose	Main side effects	Important interactions and contraindications
Flutamide	Antiandrogens	250 mg TDS	Gynecomastia, increased in liver transaminases. GI disturbances	Periodic liver function monitoring is required
Bicalutamide	Antiandrogens	50–150 mg OD	Gynecomastia, increased in liver transaminases	Periodic liver function monitoring is required
Cyproterone acetate (CPA)	Steroidal antiandrogens	100 mg TDS	Gynecomastia, increased in liver transaminases	Severe cardiovascular complications in 10%; contraindicated in people with heart failure
Goserelin	LHRH analogs	3.6 mg monthly 10.8 mg 3-monthly	Hot flashes, loss of libido, erectile dysfunction, generalized tiredness, osteoporosis, weight gain, anemia	
Leuprolin	LHRH analogs	3.75 mg monthly	Hot flashes, loss of libido, erectile dysfunction, generalized tiredness, osteoporosis, weight gain, anemia	
Abarelix	LHRH antagonists	11.25 3-monthly 113 mg monthly	Hot flashes, loss of libido, erectile dysfunction, generalized tiredness, osteoporosis, weight gain, anemia	Severe anaphylaxis
Diethyl stilbesterol	Acts by competitive inhibition with androgens at their hypothalamic receptors	1 mg OD	Severe thromboembolic phenomena. Dose reduced from 5 to 1 mg	Not given in patients with history of DVT, PE, hypercoagulability status; impaired cardiac or liver function; usually given with aspirin 75 mg OD

Ketoconazole	Adrenal antiandrogens	200 mg OD	Gynecomastia, weakness, hepatic dysfunction, visual disturbance, and nausea	Administration requires steroid supplementation to avoid adrenal insufficiency
Finasteride	5 alpha reductase inhibitors	5 mg OD	Inhibits the conversion of testosterone into DHT	No defined role in the standard care of PCa
Docetaxel	Antineoplastic agent belonging to the taxoid family that acts by disrupting the microtubular network in cells that is essential for mitotic and interphase cellular functions	75 mg/m² every 3 weeks for 10 cycles	GI disturbances, bone marrow suppression, hepatotoxicity	Incidence of treatment-related mortality associated with docetaxel therapy is increased in patients with abnormal liver function; caution with neutropenia
Zoledronic acid	An inhibitor of osteoclastic bone resorption	4 mg IV infusion over 15 min; minimum 7 days before repeat	fever; flu-like syndrome: fever, chills, bone pain and/or arthralgias, and myalgias; GI reactions	Patients with significant hypersensitivity to zoledronic acid or other bisphosphonates
Estramustine phosphate	Cytotoxic	600 mg/m²/day PO	Heme, mucositis, nausea and vomiting, edema, deep venous thrombosis	Caution in patients with impaired cardiovascular status
Prednisolone	Glucocorticoides	10 mg OD	Fluid and electrolyte disturbances, muscle weakness, osteoporosis, glucose intolerance	Systemic fungal infections and known hypersensitivity to components

Notes:

Antiandrogens: Competitive inhibitors of ligand-binding portion of the androgen receptors at the target organ

LHRH analogs: Luteinizing hormone (LH) releasing hormone agonists act by persistent stimulation of the LH receptors at the anterior pituitary, and subsequent inhibition of LH release due to down regulation of the LH receptors

LHRH antagonists: Act by blocking the LH receptors at the anterior pituitary; hence, provide rapid onset of action, avoiding the "flare" phenomenon of the initial androgen surge, commonly seen in the LHRH analogs

Adrenal antiandrogens: Decrease the synthesis of the adrenal androgens via inhibition of the Cytochrome P450 enzyme

Luteinizing Hormone-Releasing Hormone (LHRH) Agonists

The introduction of the LHRH agonists in the 1980s revolutionized the treatment of advanced PCa. Long-acting LHRH agonists (buserelin, goserelin, leuprorelin, and triptorelin) are currently the predominant forms of ADT for advanced PCa [2]. They are synthetic agonists of LHRH, generally delivered as depot injections on a 1, 2, or 3 monthly basis, which interfere with the hypothalamic–pituitary–gonadal axis. They initially stimulate the pituitary LHRH receptors, inducing a transient rise in LH and FSH release and consequently elevate testosterone production ("testosterone flare" phenomenon), which begins approximately within 2 or 3 days after the first injection, and lasts through approximately the first week of therapy [3]. This can result in a transient increase in PCa growth, hence, some patients can experience a worsening of bone pain, acute bladder outlet obstruction, obstructive renal failure and fatal cardiovascular events due to hypercoagulation status. Importantly, spinal cord compression from vertebral metastases collapse may occur resulting in fatal consequences.

Constant exposure to LHRH after treatment with an LHRH agonist, however, eventually causes down regulation of the receptors in the pituitary, inhibition of FSH and LH release, and a concomitant decrease in testosterone production. The level of testosterone decreases to castration levels usually within 2–4 weeks. In a recent meta-analysis evaluating single-therapy ADT for advanced CaP, LHRH agonists have shown comparable efficacy relative to orchiectomy and DES [4].

Concomitant therapy with an antiandrogen certainly decreases the incidence of clinical relapse, but it does not completely remove the possibility of their occurrence. Based on pharmacokinetic considerations, it is recommended that administration of antiandrogens should be started on the same day, or a few days prior to the depot injection, and treatment should be continued for a 2-week period. However, for patients with impending spinal cord compression, alternative strategies for immediately ablating testosterone levels must be considered, such as bilateral orchiectomy or LHRH antagonists.

Antiandrogens

Antiandrogens are a treatment option in some patients with PCa. However, it has to be taken into account that the hormonal effect is inferior to castration. Nonsteroidal antiandrogens competitively inhibit the binding of androgens to the androgen receptor. As a result, the serum testosterone levels are not suppressed and may even increase.

Cyproterone acetate (CPA) is a steroidal, progestational antiandrogen that blocks the androgen-receptor interaction and reduces the serum testosterone through a weak antigonadotropic action [5]. It can be used as a monotherapy or as an agent to prevent disease flare during initiation of LHRH agonist therapy. CPA can also suppress hot flashes in response to ADT with LHRH agonists or orchiectomy. Although it is generally well tolerated, CPA is also associated with a high rate of cardiovascular complications.

Antiandrogen Monotherapy in Locally Advanced or Metastatic Disease

The results obtained from the ongoing Early PCa Program after a median follow-up of 7.4 years has shown that high-dose bicalutamide has emerged as an alternative to castration for patients with locally advanced non-metastatic PCa, and highly selected, well-informed cases of metastatic PCa, but should be avoided in patients with localized PCa [6].

LHRH Antagonists

Abarelix is one of the new, modified gonadotropin-releasing hormone antagonists. Unlike the standard LHRH agonists, abarelix is a direct LHRH antagonist, and thus, avoids the flare phenomenon. This compound was recently compared with leuprolide acetate in a phase III randomized trial 29. Medical castration, as measured by the serum testosterone levels, was achieved in 75% of the abarelix group by day 15, when compared with 10% of patients in the leuprolide group.

The percentage decrease in PSA was significantly greater in the abarelix group on day 15 after treatment. At day 29, post-treatment and beyond, the PSA levels were similar between the leuprolide and abarelix groups. Owing to the lack of long-term follow-up data, it is not yet possible to determine whether abarelix and leuprolide will provide identical rates of disease control [7]

Combined Androgen Blockade

The superiority of combined androgen blockade (i.e., the combination of an antiandrogen with orchiectomy or medical castration) as the primary treatment for advanced PCa has not been proven conclusively up to date, despite a large number of randomized trials.

A meta-analysis of 20 trials found no differences between combined androgen blockade and castration when 2-year overall survival was evaluated. Based on the ten trials with the available 5-year survival data, however, this meta-analysis, did show a significant survival (25.4% vs. 23.6%) advantage for combined androgen blockade [8,9]. Combined androgen blockade using a nonsteroidal antiandrogen tends to be superior to those using CPA in delaying progression [8,9].

The limited advantage of combined treatment over mono-therapy must, however, be balanced against higher side effects and costs. The additional costs for one quality-adjusted life-year gained using combined androgen blockade over orchiectomy alone have been estimated to be $1million. Combined androgen blockade is an option for patients with advanced or metastatic PCa. It is, however, not the standard form of androgen ablative therapy for primary application [8,9].

Antiandrogen Withdrawal Syndrome and Secondary Hormonal Manipulations

Failure after initial hormonal treatment does not necessarily mean treatment refractory disease progression. Secondary hormonal manipulations are a safe and effective but short-term option in patients with failure after primary hormonal therapy [10]. When anantiandrogen is a part of the treatment regimen, discontinuation may result in the so-called antiandrogen withdrawal syndrome, described for the first time by Kelly and Scher in 1993. The incidence of this effect has been reported to be 15–20% and it lasts for 5 months on average [10]. Replacement of an initially given antiandrogen by an alternative substance may also result in a PSA response. After initial antiandrogen monotherapy, orchiectomy at the time of failure of initial treatment may lead to a PSA response and symptomatic improvement.

Second-line treatment with bicalutamide has been shown to improve symptoms and decrease pain in patients without prior antiandrogen therapy. A 50% PSA decrease has been described after second-line treatment with nonsteroidal antiandrogens in 14–50% of cases [10].

Responders to second-line hormonal treatment may be expected to survive significantly longer than nonresponders. Overall, however, it is still doubtful whether secondary hormonal manipulations do actually improve survival. However, the suppression of testicular androgens should be continued when the disease is hormone refractory, as withdrawal of treatment may decrease chance of survival [10].

Additional Treatments

Estrogen therapy was first introduced for the treatment of PCa as an alternative to bilateral orchiectomy; unfortunately, the treatment was associated with a high risk of cardiovascular complications (myocardial infarction, stroke, and pulmonary embolism), thus, limiting its use. Interest in low-dose estrogen therapy has renewed as a potential treatment that suppresses testosterone and achieves high PSA response rates, without decreasing the bone mineral density in patients with androgen-independent disease [11].

Another approach is the addition of ketoconazole, an inhibitor of steroid synthesis, following antiandrogen withdrawal. In patients showing response following antiandrogen withdrawal, the addition of ketoconazole increased the PSA response rate from 11 to 27% [12]. However, ketoconazole is associated with a number of side effects, including gastrointestinal events, fatigue, and hepatotoxicity, and its use in PCa remains investigational.

Neoadjuvant and Adjuvant Androgen Deprivation Therapy to Radiotherapy

Data from prospective randomized trials supports the use of adjuvant hormonal treatment after external beam radiotherapy [13]. High-risk patients with locally advanced disease or positive lymph nodes seem to benefit from immediate androgen deprivation after external beam radiotherapy, whereas in the earlier stages, the differences tend to diminish. The beneficial effect of adjuvant hormonal therapy in the external beam radiotherapy setting has been attributed to an elimination of occult metastases and a potential additive effect by induction of apoptosis [13]. However, the degree to which the observed survival advantages may be attributed to hormonal therapy alone is still unknown.

The role of neoadjuvant ADT to radiotherapy in patients with high-risk disease is more controversial. The Radiation Therapy Oncology Group (RTOG) 8610 trial was the first major phase III randomized trial investigating the effect of short-term neoadjuvant ADT to radiotherapy in patients with locally advanced PCa. A significant overall survival benefit was observed in patients who received radiotherapy plus neoadjuvant Zoladex, followed by adjuvant antiandrogen therapy, when compared with those who received radiotherapy alone [14].

Recently, Roach et al. demonstrated the long-term followup results of the RTOG 8610 trial, and confirmed the important clinical benefits of adding short-term neoadjuvant ADT to radiotherapy in patients with locally advanced PCa [15].

Long-Term vs. Short-Term Adjuvant Androgen Deprivation Therapy to Radiotherapy

The optimal duration of adjuvant ADT to RT remains under question. In the RTOG 9202 study, where patients who received radiotherapy with neoadjuvant hormonal therapy were randomized to receive goserelin (for 2 years) or no further androgen deprivation, there was a significant improvement in all the end points, except the overall survival with adjuvant goserelin at 5- and 10-year follow-up [16]. However, in patients who had PCa with a Gleason score of 8–10, goserelin was associated with a significant improvement in the overall survival at the 5-year follow-up.

The recently updated European Organization for Research and Treatment of Cancer (EORTC) 22961 trial showed that survival with 6-month adjuvant ADT seems to be shorter than that with 3-year adjuvant ADT after RT for patients with locally advanced PCa. Thus, neoadjuvant hormone therapy seems beneficial in carefully selected patients. As the outcome of neoadjuvant and adjuvant ADT to local treatment depends on the stage of the cancer, more studies are warranted in order to investigate the value of each of these therapies in patient populations with different disease stages [17].

Intermittent Hormone Therapy (IHT)

Although the 2005 EAU guidelines described intermittent therapy as investigational, this approach is being used in clinical practice. IHT, in which on-treatment periods are alternated with off-treatment periods, is increasingly being investigated as an alternative to continuous hormone therapy. IHT treatment aims to minimize the side effects, maintain or improve the quality of life (QoL), and delay the progression to hormone refractory prostate cancer. Several phase II trials have demonstrated the feasibility of IHT. QoL was improved during off-treatment periods, and treatment-related morbidity was reduced. Moreover, IHT did not appear to negatively influence time-to-progression or survival. Well-designed phase III trials are currently ongoing, and preliminary results confirm the benefits of IHT with respect to QoL and treatment-related morbidity. One of these studies is a Portuguese study on 626 patients who received a 3-month induction course of hormonal therapy before being randomized to either intermittent or continuous combined androgen blockade. This study recently reported that, after a median 51 months of follow-up, there was no significant difference in the overall survival or objective progression-free survival with intermittent therapy versus continuous therapy [18]. Findings from this and other studies will clarify whether this approach offers equivalent survival to continuous CAB.

Hormone Refractory or Androgen Independent PCa

This is a very heterogeneous disease including a variety of different patient cohorts with significant different median survivals. Androgen independence may be mediated through mutations of the androgen receptor gene, but our understanding of the mechanism of androgen independence still remains incomplete.

The overall effect of continued testicular androgen suppression in hormone refractory prostate cancer is minimal at best. However, in the absence of prospective data, it seems appropriate to view the modest potential benefits against the minimal risk of treatment and continue androgen suppression indefinitely in these patients.

The lack of options available for the treatment of hormone-resistant PCa presents a significant challenge to clinicians. In the TAX237 chemotherapy trial, the median overall survival rates for patients treated with docetaxel every 3 week was 18.9 months, when compared with 16.4 months for the patients in the control arm [19]. The ongoing studies on new drugs, such as satraplatin and ixabepilone, will define the role of these agents for the second-line treatment of hormone refractory prostate cancer.

Key Points

1. Androgen Deprivation Therapy (ADT) delays progression, prevents potentially catastrophic complications, and effectively palliates symptoms, but does not prolong survival, in prostate cancer (PCa).

2. In advanced PCa, all forms of castration, such as mono-therapy (orchiectomy, LHRH, and DES), have equivalent therapeutic efficacy.
3. There is considerable evidence that ADT combined with external beam radiation therapy improves overall survival, cancer-specific survival, and arrest of disease progression, although the optimal timing and duration of ADT in this combination remain undefined.
4. In advanced PCa, the addition of a nonsteroidal anti-androgen to castration (Combined Androgen Blockade) results in a small advantage in overall survival over castra-tion alone, but is associated with increased adverse events, reduced QoL, and high costs.
5. Intermittent and "minimal" ADT should still be regarded as experimental therapies.

References

1. Huggins C, Hodges CV (1941) Studies on prostatic cancer: I. The effect of castration, of estrogen and of androgen injection on serum phosphatases in metastatic carcinoma of the prostate. Cancer Res 1:293–297
2. McLeod DG (2003) Hormonal therapy: historical perspective to future directions. Urology 61(2 Suppl 1):3–7
3. Agarwal DK, Costello AJ, Peters J, Sikaris K, Crowe H (2000) Differential response of prostate specific antigen to testosterone surge after luteinizing hormone-releasing hormone analogue in PCa and benign prostatic hypertrophy. BJU Int 85(6):690–695
4. Seidenfeld J, Samson DJ, Hasselblad V, Aronson N, Albertsen PC, Bennett CL, Wilt TJ (2000) Single-therapy androgen suppression in men with advanced PCa: a systematic review and meta-analysis. Ann Intern Med 132(7):566–567
5. de Voogt HJ (1992) The position of cyproterone acetate (CPA), a steroidal anti-androgen, in the treatment of PCa. Prostate Suppl 4:91–95
6. McLeod DG, Iversen P, See WA, Morris T, Armstrong J, Wirth MP (2006) Casodex early pca trialists' group. bicalutamide 150 mg plus standard care vs standard care alone for early pca. BJU Int 97(2):247–254

7. McLeod D, Zinner N, Tomera K et al (2001) A phase 3, multi-center, open-label, randomized study of abarelix versus leupro-lide acetate in men with PCa. Urology 58:756–761

8. Samson DJ, Seidenfeld J, Schmitt B, Hasselblad V, Albertsen PC, Bennett CL et al (2002) Systematic review and metaanalysis of monotherapy compared with combined androgen blockade for pa-tients with advanced prostate carcinoma. Cancer Res 95:361–376

9. PCa Trialists' Collaborative Group (2000) Maximum androgen blockade in advanced PCa: an overview of the randomised trials. Lancet Oncol 355:1491–1498

10. Lam JS, Leppert JT, Vemulapalli SN, Shvarts O, Belldegrun AS (2006) Secondary hormonal therapy for advanced PCa. J Urol 175:27–34

11. Scherr DS, Pitts WR Jr (2003) The nonsteroidal effects of di-ethylstilbestrol: the rationale for androgen deprivation therapy without estrogen deprivation in the treatment of prostatecancer. J Urol 170:1703–1708

12. Small EJ, Halabi S, Dawson NA et al (2004) Antiandrogen with-drawal alone or in combination with ketoconazole in androgen-independent PCa patients: a phase III trial (CALGB 9583). J Clin Oncol 22:1025–1033

13. Bolla M, Collette L, Blank L et al (2002) Long-term results with immediate androgen suppression and external irradiation in pa-tients with locally advanced PCa (an EORTC study): a phase III randomised trial. Lancet 360:103–108

14. Pilepich MV, Winter K, John MJ et al (2001) Phase III Radia-tion Therapy Oncology Group (RTOG) trial 86–10 of andro-gen deprivation adjuvant to definitive radiotherapy in locally advanced carcinoma of the prostate. Int J Radiat Oncol Biol Phys 50:1243–1252

15. Roach M III, Bae K, Speight J et al (2008) Short-term neoad-juvant androgen deprivation therapy and external-beam radio-therapy for locally advanced PCa: long-term results of RTOG 8610. J Clin Oncol 26:585–591

16. Hanks GE, Pajak TF, Porter A et al (2003) Phase III trial of long-term adjuvant androgen deprivation after neoadjuvant hormonal cytoreduction and radiotherapy in locally advanced carcinoma of the prostate: the Radiation Therapy Oncology Group Protocol 92-02. J Clin Oncol 21:3972–3978

17. Bolla M, De Reijke TM, Van Tienhoven GJ, et al (2008) Six-month concomitant and adjuvant hormonal treatment with external beam irradiation is inferior to 3-years hormonal treatment for locally

advanced PCa: results of the EORTC randomised phase III trial 22961. Eur Urol Suppl 7:117, abstract 186

18. Calais Da Silva FM, Calais Da Silva F, Bono A, et al (2006) Phase III intermittent MAB vs. continuous MAB. J Clin Oncol 24:220, abstract 4513

19. Tannock IF, de Wit R, Berry WR et al (2004) Docetaxel plus prednisone or mitoxantrone plus prednisone for advanced PCa. N Engl J Med 351:1502–1512

Chapter 4
Testicular Cancer

Daniel Rottke and Peter Albers

Introduction

In almost all cases, the first step in treatment of testis cancer is surgery, usually by inguinal orchidectomy. Histological diagnosis is usually either seminomatous germ cell tumor (Seminoma) or non-seminomatous germ cell tumor (NSGCT; Non-seminoma). Clinical stage (CS) is then established with cross-sectional imaging according to the American Joint Committee on Cancer (AJCC) staging classification of tumor, node, metastases (TNM) and serum tumor markers, such as α-fetoprotein (AFP), β–human chorionic gonadotrophin (βHCG) and Lactate dehydrogenase (LDH).

Table 4.1 reviews the TNM classification, and a description of the clinical stages is presented in Table 4.2.

Stage I disease is confined to the testis, Stage II has varying degrees of retroperitoneal nodal involvement depending on the size (Stage II A, B, and C), and Stage III indicates supra-diaphragmatic and visceral metastatic disease with varying degrees of raised tumor markers. The use of tumor markers in the TNM staging is unique to testis cancer.

In cases of primary metastatic disease, induction chemotherapy is applied. The three main therapeutic agents in these cases

P. Albers (✉)
Department of Urology, University Medical Center Heinrich-Heine
University of Duesseldorf, Duesseldorf, Germany
e-mail: urologie@uni-duesseldorf.de

I.S. Shergill et al. (eds.), *Medical Therapy in Urology*,
DOI 10.1007/978-1-84882-704-2_4,
© Springer-Verlag London Limited 2010

TABLE 4.1. Tumor nodes metastasis (TNM) classification of testis cancer.

Primary tumor (T)	
TX	The primary tumor cannot be assessed
T0	There is no evidence of primary tumor
Tis	Carcinoma in situ (noninvasive cancer cells)
T1	The tumor has not spread beyond the testicle and the epididymis. Cancer cells are not found inside blood vessels or lymph vessels next to the tumor. The cancer may have grown through the inner layer surrounding the testicle (tunica albuginea) but not the outer layer covering the testicle (tunica vaginalis)
T2	Similar to T1 except that the cancer has spread to blood vessels, lymphatic vessels, or the tunica vaginalis
T3	The tumor invades the spermatic cord (which contains blood vessels, lymphatic vessels, nerves, and the vas deferens)
T4	The tumor invades the scrotum
Regional lymph nodes (N)	
NX	Regional (nearby) lymph nodes cannot be assessed
N0	No metastasis (spread) to regional lymph nodes is seen on X-rays
N1	There is metastasis in at least one lymph node, but no lymph node is larger than 2 cm (about 3/4 in.) in any dimension
N2	There is metastasis in at least one lymph node that is larger than 2 cm, but is not bigger than 5 cm (2 in.) in any dimension
N3	There is metastasis to at least 1 lymph node that is larger than 5 cm in any dimension
If the lymph nodes were taken out during surgery, there is a slightly different classification	
pNX	Regional (nearby) lymph nodes cannot be assessed
pN0	There is no metastasis to regional lymph nodes
pN1	There is metastasis (spread) to 1–5 lymph nodes, with no lymph node larger than 2 cm (about 3/4 in.) across in greatest dimension
pN2	There is metastasis in at least one lymph node that is bigger than 2 cm but not larger than 5 cm; OR metastasis to more than 5 lymph nodes that aren't bigger than 5 cm (1 in) across (in greatest dimension); OR the cancer is growing out the side of the lymph node
pN3	There is metastasis to at least one lymph node that is bigger than 5 cm
Distant metastasis (M)	
MX	Distant metastasis cannot be assessed
M0	There is no distant metastasis (no spread to lymph nodes outside the area of the tumor or other organs, such as the lungs)
M1	Distant metastasis is present
M1a	The tumor has metastasized to distant lymph nodes or to the lung
M1b	The tumor has metastasized to organs, such as liver, brain, bone, and others

TABLE 4.2.   Clinical stages of germ cell tumors (GCTs).

Clinical stages			
Stage 0	pTis	N0	M0	S0, SX
Stage I			
IA	pT1	N0	M0	S0
IB	pT2–4	N0	M0	S0
IS	Every pT/TX	N0	M0	S1–3
Stage II			
IIA	Every pT/TX	N1	M0	S0 and S1
IIB	Every pT/TX	N2	M0	S0 and S1
IIC	Every pT/TX	N3	M0	S0 and S1
Stage III			
IIIA	Every pT/TX	Every N	M1, M1a	S0 and S1
IIIB	Every pT/TX	N1–3	M0	S2
	Every pT/TX	Every N	M1, M1a	S2
IIIC	Every pT/TX	Every N	M0	S3
	Every pT/TX	Every N	M1, M1a	S3
	Every pT/TX	Every N	M1b	Every S

Notes

SX: Marker studies not available or not performed

S0: Markers normal

S1: LDH < 1, 5 × Norm and β-HCG (IU/l) < 5,000 and AFP (ng/ml) < 1,000

S2: LDH 1, 5-10 × Norm and β-HCG (IU/l) 5,000-50,000 and AFP (ng/ml) 1,000-10,000

S3: LDH > 10 × Norm and β-HCG (IU/l) > 50,000 and AFP (ng/ml) > 10,000

are cisplatin, etoposide, and bleomycine, also known as BEP- or PEB-regimen. This regimen is applied depending on the stage, in seminoma CS IIC/III (3–4 cycles), marker-positive NSGCT CS IIA/B, and NSGCT CS III. Depending on the International Germ Cell Cancer Collaborative Group (IGCCCG) risk classification (Table 4.3), 3 or 4 cycles of BEP are used. PEB is also the standard chemotherapeutic regimen in the adjuvant treatment of non-seminoma CS I with vascular invasion (2 cycles). Prognostic factors strongly influence the decision for or against adjuvant treatment in seminoma and NSGCT. With the help of a risk-adapted approach, about 50% of patients with CS I testis cancer may favor close surveillance, instead of immediate adjuvant treatment. Several well-conducted trials have helped to substantiate the management. Interestingly, surgical staging by retroperitoneal lymph node dissection (RPLND) has become

TABLE 4.3.   Prognostic factors for advanced GCTs (clinical stage IIC/III) of the International Germ Cell Cancer Collaborative Group (IGCCCG).

Good prognosis (survival rate is 90%)	
Non-seminoma	Gonadal or retroperitoneal tumor and *low markers* and no extrapulmonary organ metastases
Low markers	AFP < 1,000 ng/ml and β-HCG < 1,000 ng/ml (<5,000 IU/l) and LDH <1,5 × normal
Seminoma	Every localization of primary tumor and every marker height and no extrapulmonary organ metastases
Intermediate prognosis (survival rate is 80%)	
Non-seminoma	Gonadal or retroperitoneal tumor and *intermediate markers* and no extrapulmonary organ metastases
Intermediate markers	AFP 1,000–10,000 ng/ml or β-HCG 1,000–10,000 ng/ml (5,000–50,000 IU/l) or LDH 1,5–10 × Normal
Seminoma	Every localization of primary tumor and every marker height and *extrapulmonary organ metastases* (liver, CNS, bone, intestinum)
Poor prognosis (survival rate is 50%)	
Non-seminoma	Gonadal or retroperitoneal tumor and *extrapulmonary organ metastases or high marker* or *mediastinal non-seminoma* independent of other risk factors
High markers	AFP > 10,000 ng/ml or β-HCG > 10,000 ng/ml (>50,000 IU/l) or LDH >10 × Normal

an exception. Patients with NSGCT with high risk for occult metastatic disease may favor adjuvant chemotherapy, and in patients with seminoma, radiotherapy with reduced dosage may be challenged by carboplatin monotherapy. Ifosfamide-based regimens might be applied in second- or third-line salvage therapy.

Medical Therapies in Testicular Cancer

The specific medical therapies used in testis cancer are summarized in Table 4.4, and a general overview of the

TABLE 4.4. Medical therapies in testicular cancer.

Name	Mode of action	Drug toxic effects	Important interactions (IA) and contraindications (CI)
Cisplatin	DNA-replication inhibitor by cross-linking, alkylating agent: (1) attachment of alkyl groups to DNA bases, resulting in the DNA being fragmented by repair enzymes in their attempts to replace the alkylated bases, preventing DNA synthesis and RNA transcription from the affected DNA, (2) DNA damage via the formation of cross-links which prevents DNA from being separated for synthesis or transcription, and (3) the induction of mispairing of the nucleotides leading to mutations	Nephrotoxicity, ototoxicity, hypomagnesemia, neuropathy, infertility	IA: Plasma levels of anticonvulsant agents may become subtherapeutic during cisplatin therapy. CI: preexisting renal impairment, myelosuppressed patients, hearing impairment, history of allergic reactions to cisplatin or other platinum-containing compounds
Etoposide	DNA-replication inhibitor through Topoisomerase II – Inhibition	Secondary leukemia	IA: High-dose cyclosporin A resulting in concentrations above 2000 ng/mL administered with oral etoposide has led to an 80% increase in etoposide exposure with a 38% decrease in total body clearance of etoposide compared to etoposide alone. CI: hypersensitivity or an idiosyncratic reaction in the past
Bleomycin	DNA-replication inhibitor by cross-linking. Bleomycin is an antibiotic which has been shown to have antitumor activity. It selectively inhibits the synthesis of deoxyribonucleic acid (DNA). The guanine and cytosine content correlates with the degree of mitomycin-induced cross-linking. At high concentrations of the drug, cellular RNA and protein synthesis are also suppressed. Bleomycin has been shown in vitro to inhibit B cell, T cell, and macrophage proliferation and impair antigen presentation, as well as the secretion of interferon gamma, TNFa, and IL-2	Allergic reactions; a severe reaction consisting of low blood pressure, mental confusion, fever, chills, and wheezing; pulmonary fibrosis; Raynaud's phenomenon	IA: Certain antibiotics, cyclosporine, diuretic, foscarnet, and vaccines. CI: hypersensitivity or an idiosyncratic reaction in the past

(continued)

TABLE 4.4. (continued)

Name	Mode of action	Drug toxic effects	Important interactions (IA) and contraindications (CI)
Carboplatin	DNA-replication inhibitor by crosslinking, alkylating agent	Ototoxicity, nephrotoxicity, neuropathy, electrolyte (Ca, Mg, K, Na) disturbances, Anemia, leucopenia, allergic reactions	IA: The renal effects of nephrotoxic compounds may be potentiated by Carboplatin. CI: Carboplatin should not be employed in patients with severe bone marrow depression or significant bleeding
Ifosfamide	DNA-replication inhibitor by cross-linking, alkylating agent	Nephrotoxicity, hemorrhagic cystitis (→mesna), SIADH, central nervous system toxicity, leukopenia thrombocytopenia, anemia, Nausea, vomiting, hair loss	IA: CYP3A4 inducers may increase the levels/effects of acrolein (the active metabolite of ifosfamide). CYP3A4 inhibitors may decrease the levels/effects of acrolein. CI: Hypersensitivity to ifosfamide or any component of the formulation; patients with severely depressed bone marrow function; pregnancy
Vinblastine	Inhibition of mitosis at metaphase through its interaction with tubulin. Vinblastine binds to the microtubular proteins of the mitotic spindle, leading to crystallization of the microtubule and mitotic arrest or cell death	Constipation or ileus, SIADH	IA: Phenytoin, vinblastine sulfate, inhibitors of hepatic cytochrome P450 isoenzymes in the CYP 3A subfamily (e.g., erythromycin, doxorubicin, etoposide), hepatic dysfunction. CI: granulocytopenia, bacterial infection

chemotherapeutic regimens commonly used is presented in Table 4.5 A detailed description according to CS and histological type is discussed in the paragraph that follows.

Seminoma Clinical Stage I

About 15–20% of CS I seminoma patients have subclinical metastatic disease, usually in the retroperitoneum, and will relapse after orchidectomy alone. Tumor size >4 cm and rete testis invasion have been recognized as risk factors for occult metastatic disease. Patients with both the risk factors represent a high-risk group (recurrence rate of 32%) and should receive adjuvant radiation of the paraaortic field or alternatively single-agent carboplatin treatment. Low-risk patients (none of the risk factors, recurrence rate <10%) may be managed by surveillance as the preferred treatment option. Nevertheless, the cure rate in CS I seminoma patients is almost 100% and can be achieved with either strategy.

There seems to be no significant difference in the relapse rate, the time to relapse, and the survival rate after a median of 4-year follow-up when compared with adjuvant treatment with either radiation or one-cycle single-agent carboplatin; only the patterns of relapse differ: more retroperitoneal lymph node relapse with carboplatin vs. more pelvic lymph node relapse with adjuvant irradiation. The ease of carboplatin administration and the potential reduction of the risk for contralateral testis tumors might be a clinical advantage of carboplatin over adjuvant radiotherapy. Two courses of adjuvant carboplatin seem to further reduce the relapse rate to the order of 1–3%, but further experience and long-term observations are needed. Finally, all three treatment options for seminoma CS I result in a different relapse rate (3–4% for irradiation or adjuvant carboplatin vs. 13–20% for surveillance), but there is a final cure rate of nearly 100% of the first-line treatment approach.

Non-Seminoma Clinical Stage I

Up to 30% of NSGCT patients with CS I disease have subclinical metastases and will relapse if surveillance alone is

TABLE 4.5.   Overview of chemotherapeutic regimens in testis cancer.

Regimens	Doses	Indications
BEP (=PEB) = bleomycin, etoposide, cisplatin "5-day regimen"	Days 1–5: 100 mg/m² etoposide and 20 mg/m² cisplatin. Days 2, 8, 15: bleomycin 30 mg absolute	Most important regimen. Applied in: – seminoma CS IIB (3 cycles) – seminoma CS IIC/III good prognosis (3 cycles) – seminoma CS IIC/III interm./bad prognosis (4 cycles) – non-seminoma CS I with vasc. inv. (2 cycles) – non-seminoma CS II A/B (3 cycles) – non-seminoma CS IIC/III (4 cycles)
BEP (=PEB) = bleomycin, etoposide, cisplatin "3-day-regimen"	Days 1–2: 165 mg/m² etoposide and 50 mg/m² cisplatin. day 3: 165 mg/m² etoposide Days 2, 8, 15: bleomycin 30 mg absolute	Not recommended any more. Alternatively used in the good prognosis group of advanced testis cancer
PE (= CE) = Cisplatin, Etoposide	Days 1–5: 100 mg/m² etoposide and 20 mg/m² cisplatin.	Alternative regimen for the good prognosis group of advanced metastatic testis cancer (≤ IIC), if 3 cycles PEB are not applicable because of contraindications for bleomycin. Applied in 4 cycles
Carboplatin single agent	Day 1: carboplatin AUC 7	One cycle carboplatin as alternative to adjuvant irradiation in the high risk group of seminoma CS I
PEI (VIP) = cisplatin, etoposide, ifosfamide	Days 1–5: 75 mg/m² etoposide and 20 mg/m² cisplatin and 1,200 mg/m² ifosfamide	1. Second-line chemotherapy in case of relapse after PEB: Four cycles PEI/VIP (= salvage-chemotherapy) 2. For the poor prognosis group of advanced metastatic testis cancer, standard treatment consists of four cycles of BEP. Four cycles of VIP (=PEI) are equally effective, but cause more acute myelotoxicity and are not recommended as standard therapy, but only if bleomycin is contraindicated
VeIP = vinblastine, ifosfamide, cisplatin		Alternative regimen for second-line chemotherapy in case of relapse after PEB (=salvage chemotherapy)

applied after orchiectomy. The main predictor of relapse in CS I NSGCT is the histopathological evidence of vascular invasion by tumor cells. Patients with vascular invasion are recommended to undergo adjuvant chemotherapy with 2 cycles of cisplatin, etoposide, and bleomycin (PEB), and those without vascular invasion are recommended to undergo surveillance. Only if patients or doctors are not willing to accept the relevant risk-adapted treatment or if there are conditions against the risk-adapted treatment option, RPLND should be considered. Finally, if properly performed, surveillance is also an option for nonrisk stratified patients with NSGCT CS I. Several studies involving two courses of chemotherapy with PEB as primary treatment for high-risk patients (having about 50% risk of relapse) reported a relapse rate of only 2.7%, with very little long-term toxicity. It is important to be aware of the risk of slow-growing retroperitoneal teratomas after chemotherapy and the risk of chemoresistant cancer relapse. One course of PEB as adjuvant treatment has been tested in a randomized fashion against surgery and further data on one-course PEB have been prospectively gathered by the Swedish-Norwegian Testis Cancer Group. Thus, one course of PEB currently is under investigation vs. two courses PEB in a randomized trial.

Seminoma Clinical Stage II A/B (Metastatic Disease)

Only for patients not willing to undergo radiotherapy in Stage II B, chemotherapy with 3 cycles of PEB is considered as an alternative. The standard treatment of Stage II A/B seminoma is radiotherapy extended from the paraaortic region to the ipsilateral iliac field ("hockey-stick"), including the metastatic lymph nodes in Stage IIB.

Non-Seminoma Clinical Stage II A/B (Metastatic Disease)

In all advanced cases of NSGCT, treatment should start with initial chemotherapy, except for Stage II NSGCT disease without elevated tumor markers, which alternatively can be treated with primary RPLND or surveillance. These rare cases of Stage IIA/B without marker elevation may represent metastatic differentiated teratoma.

Stage II A/B NSGCT with elevated markers should be treated according to IGCCCG "good or intermediate prognosis" NSGCT according to marker levels (3 or 4 cycles PEB for good- and intermediate-prognosis patients, respectively, followed by residual tumor resection). About 30% of patients may not achieve a complete remission after chemotherapy and will need a residual tumor resection.

Seminoma and Non-Seminoma Clinical Stage IIC/III (Advanced Metastatic Disease)

Standard treatment for patients with a "good prognosis," according to the IGCCCG, consists of 3 cycles of PEB or, where bleomycin is contraindicated, 4 cycles of PE. Equivalent to the BEP regimen given for 5 days with EP 100 mg/m^2 and cisplatin 20 mg/m^2 each day is the BEP regimen, with etoposide 165 mg/m^2 applied during day 3 and cisplatin 50 mg/m^2 during day 2. However, the 3-day regimen has increased long-term toxicity with ototoxicity, peripheral neurotoxicity, or Raynaud`s syndrome when 4 cycles are applied; hence, the original 5-day BEP regimen remains standard treatment for 4 cycles. Therapy should be given without reduction of the doses in 22-day intervals; delaying the following chemotherapy cycle is justified only in cases of neutropenic fever which is a very rare event. Secondary prophylaxis with growth factors is recommended for the following cycles in these cases. Patients in the "intermediate-prognosis" group, according to IGCCCG, achieve a 5-year survival rate of about 80%. For these patients, 4 cycles of PEB are the standard treatment. This group may be preferentially treated in prospective trials such as the EORTC GU Group trial with PEB vs. PEB plus paclitaxel, as this group represents patients with a generally less favorable prognosis. For patients with a "poor prognosis," standard treatment consists of 4 cycles of PEB. Four cycles of PEI/VIP (cisplatin, etoposide, ifosfamide) are equally effective but more toxic, and are not recommended as standard therapy. VIP (=PEI) may be preferred to BEP to avoid possible bleomycin-induced lung injury in patients with compromised pulmonary function.

Restaging and Further Treatment

Re-evaluation of the tumor is performed by imaging investigations and determining the tumor markers after two courses of chemotherapy. If marker decline and stable or regressive disease can be observed, chemotherapy will be completed (3 or 4 cycles depending on the initial stage). In cases of marker decline, but growing metastases, resection of the tumor is obligatory after termination of induction therapy, unless in the cases of emergency according to local tumor growth. If carcinoma or immature teratoma is found in the operative specimen, 2 adjuvant cycles of conventionally dosed cisplatinum-based chemotherapy may be given for those patients in whom resection was incomplete or with vital tumor >10% of resected tissues, or for those who were classified as "poor prognosis." In cases of marker-positive tumor progression during or after first-line chemotherapy, salvage chemotherapy is given, if necessary, including surgery and radiotherapy. Most recurrences after curative therapy will occur in the first 2 years; consequently, surveillance should be most frequent and intensive during this time. Late relapses can occur beyond 5 years; annual follow-up for life may therefore be advocated. After RPLND, relapse in the retroperitoneum is rare, the most likely site of recurrence being the chest. The value of chest X-ray has been recently questioned in the follow-up of patients with disseminated disease after complete remission. CT of the chest has a higher predictive value than chest X-ray. The results of therapy are dependent on the bulk of disease; thus, an intensive strategy to detect asymptomatic disease may be justifiable. However, most patients with late relapse may present with symptoms or at least with rising markers.

Salvage Chemotherapy in Relapse/Refractory Disease

In seminoma, cisplatin-based combination salvage chemotherapy will result in long-term remissions for about 50% of the patients who relapse after first-line chemotherapy. Regimens of choice are: 4 cycles of PEI/VIP (cisplatin, etoposide, ifosfamide) or 4 cycles of vinblastin, ifosfamide, cisplatin (VeIP). Standard salvage treatment in NSGCT after first-line chemotherapy consists of 4 cycles of PEI/VIP, achieving long-term remissions in 15–40% of the patients, depending on individual risk factors (location and histology of the primary tumor, response to first line treatment, duration of remissions, and level of AFP and βHCG at relapse).

Depending on the presence of adverse prognostic factors, the results of salvage therapy after first-line cisplatin-based treatment are unsatisfactory. High-dose regimens (mostly based on etoposide and carboplatin) and dose intensification are justified approaches for patients with adverse prognostic factors (e.g., progression during first-line treatment or early after first-line). New agents such as paclitaxel, docetaxel, gemcitabine, irinotecan, and oxaliplatin have been tested in the salvage setting. Recently, paclitaxel and gemcitabine have shown to be active in the treatment of refractory GCTs; both drugs are synergistic with cisplatin. Oxaliplatin seems to have activity even in truly cisplatin-refractory patients. For patients with good performance status and adequate bone-marrow function, combination regimens of these new agents (e.g., gemcitabine plus oxaliplatin) are currently recommended, as at least a small percentage of patients may again reach long-lasting remissions. It is strongly recommended to treat recurrent patients in centers with special expertise in salvage chemotherapy regimens.

Late Toxicity of Chemotherapy in Testis Cancer

The risk of a contralateral second testicular primary tumor is dependent on the patient's age and his exposure to chemotherapy (2–5% during the first 15 years). Patients with seminoma under 30 years have the highest risk, and older men with NSGCT disease display a lower risk. The probability for the development of testis cancer is much higher in the case of biopsy-proven untreated Tis (Table 4.1) in the contralateral testis (30–70% after 7–15 years). If a biopsy of the contralateral testis has not been performed, regular examinations should be carried out in patients with risk factors (testicular maldescent, atrophy of the remaining testicle, infertility). Cases of leukemia after treatment with etoposide occur most frequently during the first decade (cumulative dose etoposide <2 g: incidence 0.6%, >2 g: incidence 2%). Late effects including cardiovascular disease and metabolic syndrome should be actively monitored and treated. Patients should be strongly encouraged to stop smoking. In 15–25% of long-term survivors, late toxicity effects including hypogonadism, nephrotoxicity, persistent neurotoxicity, Raynaud's phenomena, and ototoxicity may be recognized and should be adequately treated. Monitoring of LH, follicle-stimulating hormone, and testosterone, especially in patients with sexual problems and those experiencing involuntary infertility, is important, as there is the risk of hypogonadism (10–16%).

Key Points

1. Before the implementation of cisplatin, testis cancer cure rate was around 5%. It is now 95%.
2. Seminoma CS I high-risk patients (tumor>4 cm and rete testis invasion): adjuvant radiation of the paraaortic field or alternatively single-agent carboplatin. Low-risk patients: surveillance.
3. Non-seminoma patients CS I with vascular invasion (high risk) are recommended to undergo adjuvant chemotherapy with 2 cycles of cisplatin, etoposide, and bleomycin (PEB), and patients without vascular invasion (low risk) are recommended to undergo surveillance.
4. Standard treatment of Stage II A/B seminoma: radiotherapy extended from the paraaortic region to the ipsilateral iliac field ("hockey-stick"), including the metastatic lymph nodes in Stage IIB.
5. Patients with advanced testis cancer (Non-seminomas ≥ IIA and seminomas ≥ Stage IIC) should be preferentially treated in experienced urooncological centers. Delays in appropriate therapy are associated with more extensive disease resulting in more intensive treatment and lower cure rates.

Further Reading

1. Albers P, Albrecht W, Algaba F, Bokemeyer C, Cohn-Cedermark G, Horwich A, Laguna MP (2008) Guidelines on testicular cancer. European Association of Urology (EAU), Arnhem, The Netherlands, p 54

2. Krege S et al (2008) European consensus conference on diagnosis and treatment of germ cell cancer: a report of the second meeting of the European germ cell cancer consensus group (EGCCCG): part I. Eur Urol 53:478–496

3. Krege S et al (2008) European consensus conference on diagnosis and treatment of germ cell cancer: a report of the second meeting of the European germ cell cancer consensus group (EGCCCG): part II. Eur Urol 53:497–513

Chapter 5
Penile Cancer

Giorgio Pizzocaro

Introduction

Although penile cancer is a rare disease, it is important to appreciate that it is associated with high mortality, especially if there is a delay in presentation, and the disease becomes locally advanced or metastatic. Histologically, the commonest tumor type is squamous cell carcinoma (SCC), which has an incidence of approximately 1:100,000 men per year in developed countries. It shares similar etiology, natural history, and drug responsivity with SCC of the head and neck, female genitalia, and anal canal. HPV infection is the most common etiologic factor, while circumcision prevents SCC of the penis in nearly 100% of the cases. Usually, penile cancer arises on the epithelium of the glans, sulcus, and inner prepuce, and is classified according to the grade of differentiation into G1 (well differentiated), G2 (moderately differentiated), and G3 (poorly differentiated). The tumor nodes metastases (TNM) system is used for staging purposes (Table 5.1): in situ (Cis), exophytic (Ta), invading the lamina propria (T1), invading corpora (T2), invading urethra (T3), and invading adjacent structures (T4). SCC of the penis metastasizes mainly via the lymphatics to the regional nodes: first to the inguinal, and second to the pelvic nodes. Metastases to the higher nodes

G. Pizzocaro (✉)
Urologic Clinic 2nd, Milan University San Giuseppe Hospital, Milan, Italy

I.S. Shergill et al. (eds.), *Medical Therapy in Urology*,   63
DOI 10.1007/978-1-84882-704-2_5,
© Springer-Verlag London Limited 2010

TABLE 5.1.   2002 tumor node metastasis (TNM) classification for penile cancer.

T – Primary tumor
Tx Primary tumor cannot be assessed
T0 No evidence of primary tumor
Tis Carcinoma in situ
Ta Noninvasive verrucous carcinoma
T1 Tumor invades subepithelial connective tissue
T2 Tumor invades corpus spongiosum or cavernosum
T3 Tumor invades urethra or prostate
T4 Tumor invades other adjacent structures
N – Regional lymph nodes
Nx Regional lymph nodes cannot be assessed
N0 No evidence of lymph node metastasis
N1 Metastasis in a single inguinal lymph node
N2 Metastasis in multiple or bilateral superficial lymph nodes
N3 Metastasis in deep inguinal or pelvic lymph nodes, unilateral or bilateral
M – Distant metastases
Mx Distant metastases cannot be assessed
M0 No evidence of distant metastases
M1 Distant metastases

(para-aortic, mediastinal, and supraclavicular) are exceptionally rare, and distant spread to lung, bones, and liver is only occasional. Regarding treatment for early-stage disease, several attempts have been made to avoid penile amputation, with radiotherapy a few decades ago, and more recently, with laser and conservative surgery. Nevertheless, penile amputation cannot be avoided in patients with documented corporal cavernosa invasion, while those with corpus spongiosus invasion may be cured with glansectomy and penile resurfacing. Only patients with no more than one intranodal metastasis can be cured with surgery alone. Radical inguinal lymphadenectomy is performed, and the procedure should include the following anatomical landmarks: inguinal ligament, adductor muscle, sartorius, and the floor of the dissection should be the femoral vessels. In patients with more advanced disease, adjuvant radiotherapy was performed with severe and dangerous side effects. For the last 25 years, adjuvant chemotherapy for patients following radical lymphadenectomy for lymph node metastases, and neoadjuvant chemotherapy in patients with fixed or relapsed metastatic nodes, has provided cure in a significantly increasing population of patients with advanced disease. Adjuvant and neoadjuvant chemotherapy, combined with radical surgery, is of paramount importance today to cure patients with metastatic SCC of the penis.

Medical Therapies in Penile Cancer

SCC of the penis is only a moderately chemo-responsive cancer. Bleomycin, methotrexate, and cisplatin (BMP) have been clinically tested as single agents first, and then in a combination (multi-drug) schedule [1, 2]. Other combination chemotherapy regimens evaluated to date include Vincristine, Bleomycin and Methotrexate (VBM) [3, 4] and Cisplatin/5-Fluorouracil (PF) [4]. Recently, taxanes have been added to PF, and shown promising results [5–8]. An overview of the medical therapies (chemotherapy) used in penile cancer is presented in Table 5.2, and below is an overview of the current status of the use of chemotherapy in this disease.

Single-Agent Chemotherapy

BMP were tested sequentially at Memorial Sloan Kettering Cancer Center in New York, USA [1]. In the first series of 14 patients treated with bleomycin, three objective responses were obtained at the cost of severe lung toxicities. Responses were achieved only in patients with nodal metastases. Methotrexate, at the dosage of either 250 mg/m^2 every 2–4 weeks or 30–40 mg/m^2 weekly, was given to 13 consecutive patients. One complete and seven partial responses were achieved at the cost of severe granulocytopenia in two patients. Cisplatin was administered at the dose of 70–120 mg/m^2 every 3 weeks in these pretreated patients, and 3 of 12 evaluable patients achieved an objective response, with one complete remission. All the responders were patients previously treated with bleomycin or methotrexate.

TABLE 5.2.   Medical therapy of penile cancer.

Name	Mode of action	Dose	Main side effects	Interactions/contraindications
Vincristine (Oncovin®)	Antimitotic agent – inhibits cell division during early mitosis	1 mg i.v. on day 1 (in VBM combination)	Immunosuppression, fatigue, loss of fertility, severe constipation	Avoid in pregnancy and breast-feeding as it may cause birth defects
Bleomycin	Inhibits DNA synthesis, preventing cell division	15 mg i.v. on days 1 and 2, 6 and 24 h after vincristine (in VBM combination)	Skin changes, hair loss, fever and chills, vomiting	Cumulative pulmonary toxicity because of alveolar surfactant interaction
Methotrexate	Stops DNA synthesis by reduction of tetrahydrofolate precursors and creation of new purine and thymidine nucleotides essential in DNA synthesis	30 mg i.v. on day 3 (in VBM combination)	Bone marrow toxicity, GI disturbance, hepatotoxicity and reversible pulmonary syndrome	Avoid in pregnancy (harmful on the developing fetus) May develop acquired resistance
Cisplatin (Platinol®)	Inhibition of DNA synthesis and transcription - binds to DNA with preferential binding to the N-7 position of guanine and adenine	50 mg m² i.v. in 2 h repeated on days 1 and 2 with high volume hydration and antiemetics (in PF schedule)	Renal toxicity, nausea and vomiting, decreased levels of magnesium, potassium, and calcium, taste changes, paresthesia, birth defects	Avoid vaccinations

5-FU (Fluorouracil®)	Pyrimidine antagonist inhibits DNA synthesis by blocking the formation of normal pyrimidine nucleotides and by interfering with DNA synthesis	1,000 mg/m² in 2,000 cc half glucose and half saline in 24 h. continuous i.v. infusion on days 2–5 after cisplatin 50 mg/m² on days 1 and 2	Tiredness, nausea, diarrhea, anemia, increased tendency to bruise, mouth sores, pigmentation	Synergistic with both cisplatin and carboplatin – may cause birth defects
Paclitaxel (Taxol®) a chemical found in the yew tree. (Docetaxel: synthetic compound)	Binds to microtubules and prevents their breakdown. The chromosomes become unable to move to the opposite sides of the dividing cell. Cell division is halted and cell death is induced	120–150 mg/m² on day one in 2 h 500 cc 5% glucose solution. Alternative: Docetaxel 75 mg/m² in combination with PF (reduce 5FU 50%)		

Combination Chemotherapy

Using standard combination chemotherapy principles, three drugs were used in combination to treat 14 patients with locally advanced or metastatic penile cancer. These drugs were 200 mg/m^2 methotrexate on days 1, 8, and 15 with leucovarin rescue, 20 mg/ m^2 cisplatin and 10 mg/m^2 bleomycine on days 2–5. A 72% response rate was reported: two complete responses (one of 24+ months duration and the other of only 6 months) and eight partial remissions for an average 6 month duration, at the cost of severe toxicities, such as myelosuppression, neurotoxicity, nephrotoxicity, and pulmonary fibrosis, in most cases. Notwithstanding a negative confirmatory study by South West Oncology Group (SWOG) on 40 evaluable patients with only 32% objective responders, and 11% treatment-related mortality and 17% life-threatening toxicity in the remaining patients, BMP has remained the standard treatment for advanced penile cancer since 2006.

Adjuvant Chemotherapy

The interesting outcomes achieved with a combination of low-dose VBM in advanced squamous cell head and neck cancer encouraged Pizzocaro and Piva to use this combination therapy in patients with metastatic SCC of the penis [4], using the following schedule: Vincristine (1 mg intravenously on day 1), Bleomycin (15 mg intramuscularly 6 and 24 h after vincristine), and Methotrexate (30 mg orally on day 3). This regimen was repeated weekly for 12 weeks. In elderly patients and in patients with chronic bronchitis, only the first dose of bleomycin was administered, and methotrexate was administered on day 2.

The first five patients with fixed inguinal nodes and the 12 patients with radically resected inguinal node metastases were treated with either primary or adjuvant VBM chemotherapy. Three of the five patients with unresectable inguinal metastases achieved partial remission and could undergo surgery. Only one of the 12 patients who received adjuvant VBM relapsed after a median follow-up of 42 months. Updated results reported four relapses out of 25 patients treated with adjuvant VBM for radically resected nodal metastases in the period 1979–1990. Treatment was generally well tolerated, although fever, lung fibrosis, and skin hyperpigmentation were seen [4]. These findings compared favorably with a previous series (1964–1978) of 31 patients submitted to radical inguino-pelvic lymph-node dissection alone, whose 5-year disease-free survival was only 37%, as against 84% in the last 25 patients treated with adjuvant VBM.

A more accurate analysis of these two series allowed the identification of some risk factors in patients with metastatic nodes. In the first series of 31 patients who did not receive adjuvant chemotherapy, only the involvement of a single node was associated with good prognosis, whereas in the series of 25 patients treated subsequently with adjuvant VBM in the period 1979–1990, only bilaterality of metastases and pelvic nodes involvement remained significantly associated with poor prognosis ($p = 0.006$). None of the patients who had a single intranodal metastasis suffered relapse, regardless of the postoperative treatment (category pN1).

Starting from 1991, we administered three courses of adjuvant PF in patients with more than one nodal metastases: categories pN2-3 [4]. Chemotherapy was administered for five consecutive days with premedication with corticosteroids on day 1 and antiemetics for 5 consecutive days during a 2 l. intravenous continuous infusion of half saline and 2.5% glucose with 100 mg/m^2 cisplatin divided into two doses on days 1 and 2, and 1,000 mg/m^2 daily continuous infusion of 5-FU on days 2–5. As of the year 2000, only two out of the 30 treated patients relapsed (6.7%).

In summary and according to the European Association of Urology (EAU) guidelines, adjuvant chemotherapy (two or three courses of PF) is indicated in patients with > 1 intranodal metastasis (pN2 pN3) after radical lymphadenectomy, as survival is improved [5].

Neoadjuvant Chemotherapy for Fixed Inguinal Nodes

Between 1979 and 1990, 16 consecutive patients with fixed nodal metastases from SCC of the penis were treated with neoadjuvant chemotherapy at the National Cancer Institute in Milan [4]. The first 13 patients received 12 weekly courses of VBM combination chemotherapy. Seven of these 13 patients achieved a partial remission and underwent surgery. Only five could be resected radically. Two of the five radically resected patients were alive and disease-free after 5 and 13 years, for a total 15% disease-free survival with VBM neoadjuvant chemotherapy [4]. Of the six patients treated with PF (three previously pretreated with VBM and three with chronic bronchitis and chemotherapy-naïve), five achieved a partial remission and underwent surgery, which was radical in four patients. Three of the four radically resected patients were alive and disease-free after 3, 8, and 10 years.

During the decade 1990–1999, 25 consecutive patients with fixed, ulcerated, or relapsed nodal metastases were treated with four courses of neoadjuvant PF: 22 (88%) could undergo radical surgery and 10 (40%) are long-term survivors, confirming the above mentioned results. Recently, Joerger et al. [6] reported major tumor regression after paclitaxel and carboplatin polychemotherapy in a patient with advanced penile cancer, and Hitt et al. demonstrated the superiority of cisplatin, 5-FU, and paclitaxel over PF alone in a randomized study on SCC of the head and neck [7]. Therefore, in 2004, we started to add 120 mg/m^2 Paclitaxel to the PF combination chemotherapy in advanced penile cancer – TPF regimen [8]. Corticosteroids, antihistamines, and H2 antagonist were administered before starting paclitaxel, which was diluted in 500 mL of 5% glucose. Antiemetic drugs and glutathione were administered before cisplatin, which was preceded and followed by hydration with 1 l. half saline in 2.5% glucose containing 20 mEq potassium chloride (KCl) and 10 mEq magnesium sulfate (MgSO$_4$). Also, 1,000 mg of 5-FU was diluted in 2 l. of half saline in 2.5% glucose daily and administered as an intravenous continuous infusion for four consecutive days. Patients were monitored twice a week for possible side effects of chemotherapy. Courses were repeated every 3 week, with the first response evaluation after two courses. Five out of the first six patients were responsive to the first two courses of TPF chemotherapy. Two patients completed the four planned courses, underwent postchemotherapy surgery, and only fibrosis-necrosis was found; they are alive, as well as disease-free for over 3 years. One patient underwent surgery after two courses on account of intolerance (severe nausea and vomiting) to TPF chemotherapy. Less than 20% active tumor was found within a huge necrotic inguinal mass. The patient refused further chemotherapy and has been disease-free for over 4 years. The last two patients had a clinically apparent complete remission, refused surgery, did not present at follow-up, and died of recurrent, rapidly progressing disease 4 and 10 months later.

Bermayo et al. [9] at MD Anderson Cancer Center achieved two pathological complete remission out of two patients treated with 4–5 courses of paclitaxel carboplatin and other three pathological complete remission out of five patients treated with paclitaxel, iphosfamide, and cisplatin, while all the three patients treated with BMP chemotherapy died of the disease and suffered severe toxicity.

Even though there are few reports in the literature on patients treated with paclitaxel, it appears that adding paclitaxel to carboplatin or to PF may improve the results of PF alone in metastatic disease. Postchemotherapy surgery has been considered mandatory by all authors [6, 8, 9]. BMP chemotherapy, on the contrary, is a poorly active and very toxic treatment, which is to be abandoned in current practice [10]. In summary, as per the EAU guidelines, neo-adjuvant chemotherapy is strongly recommended in patients with unresectable or recurrent lymph node metastases [5].

Key Points

1. SCC of the penis is a loco-regional invasive disease. Distant metastases, resulting from both extraregional lymph nodes (retroperitoneum and above) or hematogenous spread are exceptionally rare.
2. Primary radical surgery in advanced disease is both mutilating and followed by frequent relapses.
3. Radiotherapy is followed by frequent complications and cannot cure advanced lymph node metastases.
4. Following the concept that SCC of the head and neck, penis, female genitalia, and anal canal have the same histology,

natural history, clinical behavior, and responsiveness to chemotherapy, the treatment of these types of cancers with the same conceptual philosophy seems justified.

5. Introduction of the same chemotherapy schedules that had documented activity in SCC of the head and neck, made it possible to significantly improve the cure rate of penile cancer patients in both the adjuvant and neoadjuvant setting.

References

1. Ahmed T, Sklaroff R, Yagoda A (1984) Sequential trials of methotrexate, cisplatin and bleomycin for penile cancer. J Urol 132:465–468

2. Dexeus FH, Logothetis CJ, Sella A et al (1991) Combination chemotherapy with methotrexate, bleomycin and cisplatin for advanced squamous cell carcinoma of the male genital tract. J Urol 146:1284–1287

3. Pizzocaro G, Piva L (1988) Adjuvant and neoadjuvant vincristine, bleomycin, and methotrexate for inguinal metastases from squamous cell carcinoma of the penis. Acta Oncol 27:823–824

4. Pizzocaro G, Piva L, Bandieramonte G, Tana S (1997) Up-to-date management of carcinoma of the penis. Eur Urol 32:5–15

5. Hitt R, López-Pousa A, Martínez-Trufero J (2005) Phase III study comparing cisplatin plus fluorouracil to paclitaxel, cisplatin, and fluorouracil induction chemotherapy followed by chemoradiotherapy in locally advanced head and neck cancer. J Clin Oncol 23:8636–8645

6. Bermejo C, Busby JE (2007) Spiess PE neoadjuvant chemotherapy followed by aggressive surgical consolidation for metastatic penile squamous cell carcinoma. J Urol 177:1335–1338

7. Joerger M, Warzinek T (2004) Klaeser B major tumor regression after paclitaxel and carboplatin polychemotherapy in a patient with advanced penile cancer. Urology 63:778–780

8. Pizzocaro G, Nicolai N, Milani A (2009) Taxanes in combination with cisplatin and fluorouracil for advanced penile cancer: preliminary results. Eur Urol 55:546–551

9. Hakenberg OW, Nippgen JB, Froehner M et al (2006) Cisplatin, methotrexate and bleomycin for treating advanced penile carcinoma. BJU Int 98:1225–1227

10. http://www.uroweb.org/fileadmin/tx_eauguidelines/2009/Full/Penile_Cancer.pdf

Chapter 6
LUTS/Benign Prostatic Hyperplasia

Katie Moore and Jay Khastgir

Introduction

Terminology

As the terminology in Benign Prostatic Hyperplasia (BPH) can be very confusing, there has been a recent drive to correctly define the terms in this field of urology (Table 6.1). For the purposes of this chapter, we will refer to lower urinary tract symptoms (LUTS) resulting from benign prostate enlargement (BPE) suggestive of BPH, as LUTS/BPH. Importantly, the previously used term "prostatism" is outdated, nonspecific, and should not be used for such patients any more.

Anatomy, Physiology, and Pathology of Prostate Relevant to LUTS/BPH

The prostate gland sits at the base of the bladder and is composed of epithelial and stromal elements. The epithelial component is composed of organized acinar glands which make up a ductal system that drains into the urethra. The fibromus-

K. Moore (✉)
Department of Urology, Morriston Hospital ABM University Hospitals
NHS Trust, Swansea, UK
e-mail: katiemoore@doctors.org.uk

I.S. Shergill et al. (eds.), *Medical Therapy in Urology*,
DOI 10.1007/978-1-84882-704-2_6,
© Springer-Verlag London Limited 2010

TABLE 6.1.   Current terminology in benign prostate disease.

Term	Description	Definition
LUTS	Lower urinary tract symptoms	Non-specific term for symptoms which may be attributable to lower urinary tract dysfunction. The two main groups of LUTS are Storage LUTS (previously called irritative symptoms) and Voiding LUTS (previously called obstructive symptoms)
BPH	Benign prostatic hyperplasia	Histological basis for a diagnosis of BPE leading to BOO that results in LUTS
BOO	Bladder outflow obstruction	Urodynamically proven obstruction to passage of urine
BPE	Benign prostate enlargement	The clinical finding of an enlarged prostate, assumed to be due to BPH
BPO	Benign prostatic obstruction	BOO caused by BPE
OAB	Overactive bladder	Symptom syndrome of urgency, with or without urgency incontinence, usually accompanied by urinary frequency and nocturia

cular stromal element is composed of smooth muscle that interacts with the epithelial component. Morphologically, the prostate is divided into distinct zones, namely, transition zone (5%), central zone (25%), peripheral zone (70%), and anterior fibromuscular stroma (<1%). The transition zone is the site of the development of BPH. Proliferation of the prostatic tissue causes BOO, which usually manifests clinically as LUTS, OAB, incomplete bladder emptying, and occasionally as acute urinary retention (AUR).

There is a static and dynamic component to the development of BOO from LUTS/BPH. The static component is mediated by the volume effect of BPH. There is an increase in epithelial and stromal cell numbers (hyperplasia) in the periurethral area of the prostate. The increase in prostate cell number could reflect either proliferation of stromal and epithelial cells, impairment of programmed cell death, or both. In early BPH, cell proliferation occurs rapidly. In the later stages, cell proliferation slows down, and there is impairment of apoptosis (androgens and estrogens actively inhibit cell death). In the dynamic component, prostatic smooth muscle constriction is mediated by α1-adrenoreceptors. Smooth muscle accounts for approximately 40% of the area density of the hyperplastic prostate and contracts following administration of α adrenergic agonists. This effect is the rationale for α blocker treatment in symptomatic LUTS/BPH causing BOO.

Dihydrotestosterone (DHT) is the main intracellular androgen involved in the regulation of prostatic growth. It is formed by the action of the enzyme 5α reductase on testosterone. Testosterone diffuses into the prostate stromal and epithelial cells. In the epithelial cells, it binds directly to the androgen receptor. In the prostate stromal cells, a small proportion binds directly to the androgen receptor, but the majority binds to 5α reductase on the nuclear membrane, is converted to DHT, and then binds (with a greater affinity and therefore, a greater potency than testosterone) to the androgen receptor in the stromal cells. The androgen receptor/testosterone or androgen receptor/DHT complex then binds to specific binding sites in the nucleus, inducing transcription of androgen dependant genes and triggering a sequence of events to take place in the cell that eventually lead to cell replication. There are two isoforms of 5α reductase, type I found outside the prostate and type II found on the nuclear membrane of prostatic stromal cells but not prostatic epithelial cells.

Importantly, the severity of symptoms and bother (affect on quality of life) directs the need for treatment. Those with moderate to severe symptoms and high bother score need some form of therapy. After assessment of the patients including symptoms score, digital rectal examination and flow rates, medical therapy can be initiated. This usually takes the form of an alpha blocker (AB) or a 5α reductase inhibitor (5ARI). Recent data has also suggested the additional and safe use of anticholinergic (Ach) medication for overactive bladder (OAB) symptoms.

Assessment of LUTS/BPH Relevant to Medical Management

Several authorities worldwide have developed guidelines on the assessment, therapy, and follow-up of men suffering from LUTS/BPH (Fig. 6.1). The important aspects of the assessment

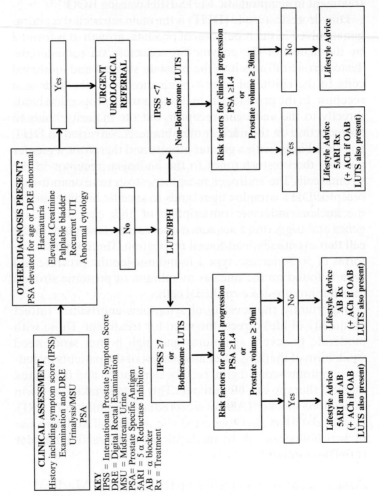

FIGURE 6.1.   Assessment and medical therapy of LUTS/BPH.

which are relevant to medical management are now discussed. First, it is important to exclude other causes of LUTS such as prostate cancer, urinary tract stones, urethral stricture, and bladder cancer, through a detailed assessment (Fig. 6.1). Once it is established that LUTS are resulting from BPE suggestive of BPH (LUTS/BPH), symptom severity should be established. This can be objectively assessed using validated questionnaires such as the International Prostate Symptom Score (IPSS), which also includes a quality of life score (Table 6.2). The IPSS is not only useful in initial stratification of symptoms (mild, moderate, or severe), but can be used to assess response to medical therapies. Generally, a 2-point improvement is regarded as clinically meaningful to patients [1]. Other important objective indicators of BOO and factors that can be used clinically to assess response to medical treatments include maximum urinary flow rate (Qmax), post void residual volume (PVR), prostate volume, and prostate specific antigen (PSA).

Finally, risk factors for the clinical progression of LUTS/BPH should be identified, namely prostate volume (≥30 mL) and PSA (≥1.4 ng/mL). Clinical progression of LUTS/BPH can be defined as worsening of symptom score, above baseline, of ≥4 points, acute urinary retention, urinary incontinence, renal insufficiency, or recurrent urinary tract infection [2].

Medical Therapies in LUTS/BPH

Several important randomized, placebo-controlled multi-centre trials have provided useful information on the effects of medical treatment for LUTS/BPH. Medical treatments are summarized in Table 6.3, and include α-blockers (AB), 5α reductase inhibitors (5ARI), as well as ACh medication.

α Blockers

Randomized, placebo-controlled multicentre trials have shown that AB demonstrate an early onset of action and lasting improvement in both symptom score and flow rates.

TABLE 6.2.   The International Prostate Symptom Score (IPSS).

	Not at all	Less than 1 time in 5	Less than half the time	About half the time	More than half the time	Almost always	Your score
Incomplete emptying Over the past month, how often have you had a sensation of not emptying your bladder completely after you finish urinating?	0	1	2	3	4	5	
Frequency Over the past month, how often have you had to urinate again less than two hours after you finished urinating?	0	1	2	3	4	5	
Intermittency Over the past month, how often have you found you stopped and started again several times when you urinated?	0	1	2	3	4	5	
Urgency Over the last month, how difficult have you found it to postpone urination?	0	1	2	3	4	5	
Weak stream Over the past month, how often have you had a weak urinary stream?	0	1	2	3	4	5	

	0	1	2	3	4	5	Your score
Straining Over the past month, how often have you had to push or strain to begin urination?	0	1	2	3	4	5	
	None	1 time	2 times	3 times	4 times	5 times or more	Your score
Nocturia Over the past month, how many times did you most typically get up to urinate from the time you went to bed until the time you got up in the morning?	0	1	2	3	4	5	
Total IPSS score							
Quality of life due to urinary symptoms	Delighted	Pleased	Mostly satisfied	Mixed – about equally satisfied and dissatisfied	Mostly dissatisfied	Unhappy	Terrible
If you were to spend the rest of your life with your urinary condition the way it is now, how would you feel about that?	0	1	2	3	4	5	6

Total score: 0–7 mildly symptomatic; 8–19 moderately symptomatic; 20–35 severely symptomatic

TABLE 6.3.   Medical therapies in LUTS/BPH.

Name	Mode of action	Oral dosage	Main side effects	Important contraindications and interactions
Alfuzosin	Selective α-blockade of α1a receptors in the prostate and bladder neck causing smooth muscle relaxation and improved urine flow.	10 mg	Postural hypotension, headache, dizziness, abnormal ejaculation	Contraindications – hypersensitivity to drug, severe hepatic impairment Potential interaction – β-blocker – increased orthostatic effects
Tamsulosin	Selective α-blockade of α1a receptors in the prostate and bladder neck causing smooth muscle relaxation and improved urine flow	400 mcg	Postural hypotension, headache, dizziness, abnormal ejaculation	Contraindications – hypersensitivity to drug, severe hepatic impairment Potential Interaction – β-blocker – increased orthostatic effects, caution in cataract surgery – floppy iris syndrome
Doxazosin	Inhibits α1-receptors causing vasodilatation and relaxation of the smooth muscle of the prostate and bladder neck	1 mg titrating to maximum of 8 mg	Postural hypotension, headache, dizziness, abnormal ejaculation	Contraindications – hypersensitivity to drug Potential Interaction – β-blocker – increased orthostatic effects
Indoramin		20 mg BD increasing to maximum 100 mg in divided dose		

Drug	Dose	Mechanism	Side effects	Notes
Prazosin	500 mcg BD increasing to maximum 2 mg BD		Postural hypotension, dizziness, parasthesia, arthralgia	
Terazosin	1 mg nocte increasing to maximum 10 mg		Postural hypotension, dizziness, weight gain, parasthesia, dyspnea	
Finasteride	5 mg OD	Inhibits 5α reductase, thus inhibiting metabolism of testosterone leading to reduction of prostate size. Onset of action 3–6 months	Impotence, decreased libido, ejaculation disorders, breast tenderness and enlargement	Decreases serum PSA levels. Should not be handled by pregnant women. Excreted in semen
Dutasteride	500 mcg OD	Inhibits 5α reductase, thus inhibiting metabolism of testosterone leading to reduction of prostate size. Onset of action 2–6 months	Impotence, decreased libido, ejaculation disorders, breast tenderness and enlargement	Contraindicated in severe hepatic impairment. Decreases serum PSA levels. Should not be handled by pregnant women. Excreted in semen

(Alfuzosin, Finasteride, and combination in the treatment of BPH), 1,000 men were randomized to alfuzosin, finasteride, or a combination. At 6 months, the improvement in IPSS was not significantly different in the alfuzosin group, when compared with the combination group. The downfall of these studies was that prostate size was below the 40 mL cut-off that finasteride had been shown to show significant improvement. Also, the follow-up period was for 1 year only.

However, the Medical Therapy of Prostatic Symptoms (MTOPS) Study, a multicentre, randomized, placebo-controlled double-blind study with 3,047 men, showed that the combination of doxazosin and finasteride was more effective than monotherapy in preventing progression of BPH and improving LUTS and urinary flow. Progression of BPH was defined as worsening of symptom score by four or more, or complications such as UTI or AUR. Doxazosin (39%) and finasteride (34%) produced similar reductions in the risk of progression, when compared with the placebo, whereas combination therapy produced a much more significant reduction (67%) in the long term. When comparing each individual arm, finasteride and combination therapy were equally effective in preventing acute urinary retention, whereas doxazosin postponed the time to occurrence of AUR. Similarly, finasteride and combination therapy significantly reduced the occurrence of an invasive procedure, whereas doxazosin delayed the occurrence of an invasive procedure. Prostate volume increased in the placebo and doxazosin groups by an average of 4.5% per annum, while in the finasteride group, there was a mean reduction of 13% and 16% in the dual therapy group. Combination therapy was shown to be well tolerated in the average man. Emphasis was placed on the fact that combination therapy had beneficial effects over the long term [2].

Combination Therapy – α Blockers and ACh Medication

A significant number of patients experience OAB symptoms as part of LUTS/BPH. As such, the TIMES study (tolterodine and tamsulosin in men with LUTS including OAB) was conducted, in which 879 patients with mixed (storage and voiding) LUTS were randomized to receiving placebo, tamsulosin alone, extended-release tolterodine alone, or tolterodine and tamsulosin in combination [11]. This trial demonstrated that combination treatment with the AB and ACh was significantly more effective than placebo or monotherapy alone. At 12 weeks, 80% of the patients receiving combination therapy reported a treatment benefit, when compared with 62% of those receiving placebo (p <0.001). The single treatments were not significantly more effective than placebo, with only 71% of patients taking tamsulosin, and 65% of those taking tolterodine reporting an improvement in symptoms. Subsequently, further analysis of this data with regard to daytime and nocturnal micturition related to urgency episodes and their severity, and to measures of quality of life, confirmed that patients on combination therapy had a significantly better outcome than those taking any of the monotherapies [12].

Management Algorithm for Medical Treatment of LUTS/BPH

The main aim of medical therapy in LUTS/BPH is to improve bothersome LUTS, restore an acceptable quality of life, and to identify patients at risk of disease progression in order to avoid an unfavorable outcome, such as acute urinary retention. As such, the algorithm in Fig. 6.1 is used for the medical therapy of LUTS/BPH, and is adapted from the British Association of Urological Surgeons (BAUS) algorithm for the management of LUTS in primary care [13]. AB are used to improve symptoms per se, especially if they are moderate/severe or bothersome, affecting quality of life. Preventative treatment, in the form of 5ARI, should be started as early as possible in patients with risk factors for clinical progression (PSA≥1.4 or Prostate volume ≥30 mL). Combination treatment (AB and 5ARI) is recommended in those symptomatic patients at risk for clinical progression, and finally, combination therapy (ACh and AB) can be reserved for patients who have troublesome OAB symptoms as well as LUTS/BPH (Fig. 6.1).

Key Points

1. Medical therapy is an established treatment for men with symptoms of LUTS/BPH.
2. α-blockers rapidly improve BPH-related symptoms and urinary flow rates, but can cause postural hypotension and dizziness.
3. 5α Reductatse Inhibitors shrink the prostate by approximately 20%, increasing flow rate and decreasing BPH progression.
4. Combination therapy of α-blockers and 5α Reductatse Inhibitors is clinically effective and beneficial, when compared with monotherapy, especially in those at risk of clinical progression, but it may be associated with a higher risk of adverse events.
5. Combination therapy of α-blockers and Anti-cholinergic medication is significantly more effective than placebo or monotherapy alone, especially in patients with overactive bladder symptoms.

References

1. Barry NJ, Fowler FJ, O' Leary MP et al (1992) The American urological association symptom index for benign prostatic hyperplasia. J Urol 148:1549–1557
2. McConnell JD, Roehborn CG, Bautista OM (2003) The long term effects of doxazosin, finasteride, and combination therapy on the clinical progression of benign prostatic hyperplasia. N Engl J Med 349:2387–2398
3. Kirby RS, Pool JL (1997) Alpha adrenoreceptor blockade in the treatment of benign prostatic hyperplasia: past, present and future. Br J Urol 80:521–532
4. Van Kerredroeck P, Jardin A, Laval KU, van Caugh P, ALFORTI Study Group (2000) Efficacy and safety of a new prolonged release formulation of the alfuzosin 10 mg once daily versus alfuzosin 2.5 mg thrice daily and placebo in patients with symptomatic benign prostatic hyperplasia. Eur Urol 37:306–313

5. JE Edwards, Moore RA (2202) Finasteride in the treatment of clinical benign prostatic hyperplasia: a systematic review of randomised trials. BMC Urol 14

6. McConnell JD, Bruskewitz R, Walsh P, Andriole G, Lieber M, Holtgrewe HL, Albertsen P, Roehborn CG, Nickel JC, Wang DZ, Taylor AM, Waldstreicher J (1998) The effect of finasteride on the risk of acute urinary retention and the need for surgical treatment among men with benign prostatic hyperplasia. finasteride long-term efficacy and safety study group. N Eng J Med 338:557–563

7. Thompson IM, Phyllis J, Goodman MS, Tangen CM et al (2003) The influence of finasteride on the development of prostate cancer. NEJM 349(3):213–222

8. Debruyne F, Barkin J, van Erps P, Reis M, Tammela TLJ, Roehrborn C (2004) Efficacy and safety of long-term treatment with the dual 5á-reductase inhibitor dutasteride in men with symptomatic benign prostatic hyperplasia. Eur Urol 46:488–495

9. Lepor H, Williford WO, Barry MJ, Brawer MK, Dixon CM, Gormley G et al (1996) The efficacy of terazosin, finasteride or both in benign prostatic hyperplasia. Veterans affairs cooperative studies benign prostatic hyperplasia study group. N Engl J Med 335(8):533–539

10. Kirby RS, Altwein JE, Bartsch G et al (1999) Results of the PREDICT (prospective european doxazosin and combination therapy) trial. J Urol 148:1467–1474

11. Kaplan SA, Roehrborn CG, Rovner ES, Carlsson M, Bavendam T, Guan Z (2006) Tolterodine and tamsulosin for treatment of men with lower urinary tract symptoms and overactive bladder: a randomized controlled trial. JAMA 296:2319

12. Rovner Eric S, Kreder K, Sussman David O, Kaplan Steven A, Carlsson M, Bavendam T, Zhonghong G (2008) Effect of tolterodine extended release with or without tamsulosin on measures of urgency and patient reported outcomes in men with lower urinary tract symptoms. J Urol 180(3):1034–1041

13. Speakman MJ, Kirby RS, Joyce A, Abrams P, Pocock R (2004) Guideline for the primary care management of male lower urinary tract symptoms. BJU Int 93(7):985–990

Chapter 7
Overactive Bladder and Incontinence

Vinay Kalsi, Abdul Chowdhury, and Kim Mammen

Introduction

Urinary incontinence (UI) is defined by the International Continence Society as "a complaint of any involuntary loss of urine." It is an extremely common condition with a suggested prevalence of more than one in three adults over the age of 40 years, having clinically significant symptoms. The condition worsens with increasing age, causing significant distress, besides having a negative impact on the patients' quality of life through a loss of dignity and an imposition of limitations on lifestyles. Despite this, UI is very much under-reported because of the perceived antisocial and embarrassing nature of this complaint. This may have considerable financial implications, and The Continence Foundation has estimated a total cost of more than £420 million for the United Kingdom (UK) (approximately 1/120th of the total expenditure of the NHS).

Classification and Terminology

Recently, there has been an active attempt to accurately define the various terms related to UI (Table 7.1). This is important as it helps to diagnose a particular condition, and also leads to

V. Kalsi (✉)
Department of Urology, Guys and st. Thomas Hospital, London, UK
e-mail: vinay.kalsi@btinternet.com

I.S. Shergill et al. (eds.), *Medical Therapy in Urology*,
DOI 10.1007/978-1-84882-704-2_7,
89

TABLE 7.1.   Definitions of terminology in overactive bladder and urinary incontinence.

Overactive bladder syndrome	A symptom syndrome of urgency with or without incontinence usually accompanied by urinary frequency and nocturia, in the absence of pathological (e.g., UTI, Stones, Bladder tumor) and metabolic factors (e.g., diabetes)
Urgency	A sudden and compelling desire to pass urine that cannot be deferred
Urge urinary incontinence (UUI)	Involuntary leakage of urine accompanied by or immediately preceded by urgency. Usually represents a severe form of overactive bladder syndrome
Stress urinary incontinence (SUI)	Involuntary leakage of urine on effort or exertion, or on coughing or sneezing
Mixed urinary incontinence	Involuntary leakage of urine associated with urgency and also with exertion, effort, sneezing, and coughing

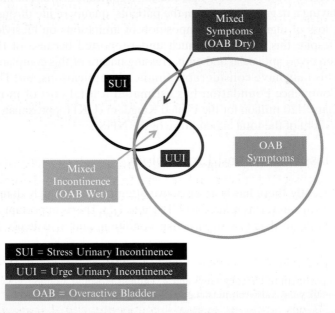

FIGURE 7.1.   Complex inter-relationship between overactive bladder (OAB), Urge Urinary Incontinence (UUI) and Stress Urinary Incontinence (SUI).

effective and appropriate treatment, as well as improved communication between various health care providers and researchers. Figure 7.1 explains the complex interrelationship between overactive bladder (OAB), urge urinary incontinence (UUI), and stress urinary incontinence (SUI).

Anatomy and Physiology of Bladder Dysfunction

The medical therapies commonly used in the management of OAB are typically competitive antimuscarinic receptor antagonists. As such, they are commonly termed anticholinergic (ACh) drugs. Although there are five types of muscarinic receptors throughout the human body (M1–M5), the detrusor muscle contains only M2 and M3 subtypes. M2 accounts for 70–80% of the receptors, but it is the remaining 20–30% of M3 receptors that seem to be the functional receptors involved in inducing a detrusor contraction. Importantly, with regard to the potential side effects, clinically relevant muscarinic receptors are present in the salivary glands (M1, M3), central nervous system, (M1, M2), the eye (M3, M5), and the heart (M2).

Clinical Assessment

The basic assessment of patients requires a history, thorough physical examination, and appropriate investigations, with the following aims of assessment:

1. Is incontinence long-standing or transient? This is because transient UI may be related to a treatable isolated event
2. Is there any underlying medical condition that may be causing the incontinence? Clearly, standard medical management will be futile, if there is an underlying treatable cause
3. Is there any voiding dysfunction causing overflow incontinence? This may suggest a complex clinical problem, which may not be treatable solely with medical management
4. Is this stress or urgency incontinence, and if there are mixed symptoms, which is the most distressing symptom? The most distressing symptoms are usually dealt with first

5. What is the effect on Quality of life? Clearly, improvement in quality of life is one of the most important aims of medical management

Conservative Management

For OAB, UUI, and SUI, certain preventative lifestyle changes are recommended. These include modifying low or high fluid intake, weight loss, especially if body mass index is >30, reduction in smoking, caffeine, and alcohol intake, ensuring a balanced diet, and avoiding constipation, as chronic straining while passing stool may be a risk factor for pelvic organ prolapse and UI. Finally, bladder training (also described as bladder re-training, bladder drill, bladder re-education, bladder discipline) lasting for a minimum of 6 weeks should be offered as first-line treatment to women with OAB, UUI, and mixed UI. Bladder training involves actively teaching the patient distraction techniques, timed voiding, and suppressing the urge to void, in an attempt to increase the interval between the desire to void and the actual void, as well as increasing the volume voided. There is good evidence that bladder training is an effective treatment for OAB, UUI, and mixed UI, with few adverse effects and low relapse rates [1].

Medical Therapies in Overactive Bladder and Incontinence

Antimuscarinic (Anticholinergic) Therapies

The medical therapies commonly used in the first-line management of OAB are competitive antimuscarinic receptor antagonists (Table 7.2), also termed ACh drugs. The detrusor muscle contains only M2 and M3 receptors, with the M3 receptors seeming to be the functionally important subtype. ACh do not inhibit the normal voiding phase of the micturition cycle, but reduce the ability of bladder muscle to contract, and in addition, alter bladder sensation and bladder capacity. Clinically, this manifests as reduced episodes

TABLE 7.2.   Medical therapies in overactive bladder (OAB) and incontinence. Important contraindications.

Name	Mode of action	Dose	Main side effects	Important interactions and contraindications
Tolterodine tartrate (Detrusitol)	Nonselective antimuscarinic receptor antagonist	2 mg BD	Dry mouth, cognitive dysfunction, blurred vision, tachycardia and constipation	Untreated closed angle glaucoma, partial or complete bowel obstruction, paralytic ileus, intestinal atony, severe colitis, myasthenia gravis, unstable cardiovascular status in acute hemorrhage
Tolterodine tartrate XL (Detrusitol XL)	Nonselective antimuscarinic receptor antagonist	4 mg OD	As above	As above
Trospium chloride (Regurin)	Nonselective antimuscarinic receptor antagonist	20 mg BD	As above	As above
Oxybutynin chloride (Ditropan)	Nonselective antimuscarinic receptor antagonist	2.5–5 mg BD to QDS (max. 20 mg in a day)	As above	As above
Oxybutynin chloride XL (Lyrinel XL)	Nonselective antimuscarinic receptor antagonist	5–30 mg OD	As above	As above
Solifenacin (Vesicare)	Selective muscarinic M2 and M3 receptor antagonist	5 mg–10 mg OD	As above	As above

(continued)

TABLE 7.2.   (continued)

Name	Mode of action	Dose	Main side effects	Important interactions and contraindications
Darifenacin (Emselex)	Selective muscarinic M3 receptor antagonist	7.5–15 mg OD	As above	As above
Propiverine hydrochloride (Detrunorm)	Nonselective anti-muscarinic receptor antagonist	15 mg OD	As above	As above
Propantheline (Pro-Banthine)	Nonselective anti-muscarinic receptor antagonist	15 mg TDS	As above	As above
Fesoterodine (Toviaz)	Antimuscarinic which bypasses the first-pass gastrointestinal and hepatic metabolism, increasing the bio-availability of the active metabolite N-desethyloxybutynin (N-DEO)		As above	As above
Oxybutynin transdermal patch (Kentera)		One patch 3.9 mg applied twice weekly (every 3–4 days)	As above Application site reaction	As above

| Duloxetine (Yentreve) | Combined norepi-nephrine and serotonin reuptake inhibitor | 40 mg twice daily | Nausea, somnolence, insomnia, dizziness | Contraindicated in patients taking MAOIs

Use with caution when taken in combination with other centrally acting drugs |

Key
OD – once daily
BD – twice daily
TDS – three times daily
QDS – four times daily
XL – extended life

of frequency, less incontinence, and increased voided volume. Data from several meta-analyses confirm these clinical observations.

In the first of these reports in 2005, data from 32 Randomised Controlled Trials (RCTs) consisting of almost 7,000 patients showed that ACh drugs decreased leaks, decreased voids, and increased cystometric capacity, in comparison to placebo; findings which were all statistically significant [2]. The main criticism, however, was that the outcomes reported (less leaks, less voids, and increased cystometric capacity) were not likely to be clinically relevant to patients. For example, even though statistically significant, a reduction of voiding episodes from 12 (placebo) to 10 (ACh drugs) may not actually denote a clinically significant difference for the patient. Furthermore, health-related quality of life (HRQL) was not included, and the ACh were all considered together, rather than individually.

Subsequently, in 2005, a systematic review and meta-analysis was published, evaluating the tolerability, safety, and efficacy of ACh drugs in OAB. In this report, an attempt was made to identify any differences between individual ACh drugs. Data from 56 trials between 1966 and 2004 were included. First, the ACh were found to be safe and efficacious, and all of them, except oxybutynin immediate release, were found to be well tolerated. Dry mouth was the most commonly reported adverse event, and no drug was associated with an increase in any serious adverse event. There were significant differences between the ACh with regard to the rates of withdrawal and the rates and range of adverse events and efficacy outcomes. The conclusion from this systematic review and meta-analysis was that ACh drugs have different tolerability and safety profiles, which are clinically significant [3].

This systematic review was updated in 2008, including data on a newly licensed ACh drug (fesoterodine). The primary aim of this study was to systematically review the evidence on the efficacy of licensed administration of ACh treatments in OAB from RCTs. Secondary aims were to review the evidence on tolerability and safety, as well as health-related quality of life. In this report, 83 studies were reviewed, and it was concluded that ACh are efficacious, safe, and well-tolerated treatments that improve HRQL. Profiles of each drug and dosage differ, and should be considered in making treatment choices [4]. Specifically, ACh were found to be more efficacious than placebo, and tolerability was found to be good, with few of the ACh having significantly higher withdrawal rates when compared with the placebo. In addition, no serious adverse event for any product was statistically significant when compared with the placebo. Improvements were seen in HRQL with treatment by darifenacin, fesoterodine, oxybutynin transdermal delivery system, propiverine extended release (ER), solifenacin, tolterodine ER and immediate release, and trospium [4].

Importantly, with regard to potential side effects, clinically relevant muscarinic receptors are also present in the salivary glands (M1, M3), Central nervous system, (M1, M2), the eye (M3, M5), and the heart (M2). The latest systematic review and meta-analysis suggested that the commonest side effect was dry mouth (29.6% on treatment vs. 7.9% on placebo) [4]. In clinical practice, other commonly seen side effects are cognitive dysfunction, blurred vision, tachycardia, and constipation (Table 7.2).

Importantly, contraindications to ACh medications include untreated closed angle glaucoma, partial or complete obstruction of the gastrointestinal tract, paralytic ileus, intestinal atony of the elderly or debilitated patient, megacolon, toxic megacolon complicating ulcerative colitis, severe colitis, and myasthenia gravis.

In current clinical practice, it appears that solifenacin and tolterodine are the main ACh drugs used. When these two drugs were directly compared in a large clinical trial (STAR trial), Solifenacin, with a flexible dosing regimen, showed greater efficacy when compared with tolterodine in decreasing urgency episodes, incontinence, urge incontinence and pad usage, and increasing the volume voided per micturition [5]. The side effects were low and comparable in both the drugs. Hence, more and more hospitals have now adopted Solifenacin as their first-line ACh based on its efficacy.

However, it should be remembered that this data has not been reproduced in other studies to date.

Botulinum Toxin

One of the most significant advances in the management of OAB and UUI recently, has been the use of injection of Botulinum Toxin A (BTX-A) directly into the smooth muscle of the detrusor, resulting in a significant improvement in neurogenic bladder dysfunction [6]. Botulinum toxin is a neurotoxin derived from *Clostridium botulinum*. Although there are seven such toxins (A to G), BTX-A is the most potent and long-acting toxin, and it blocks the presynaptic release of parasympathetic ACh-mediating detrusor contraction.

The toxin can be injected under local anesthesia using a minimally invasive technique with a flexible cystoscope, a procedure which is safe and well tolerated. The benefits of this treatment appear to exceed those expected from an agent that merely paralyzes the detrusor, and the effects last for an average of 10 months. The results of repeated injections demonstrate similar beneficial effects; the duration of action of the treatment is also comparable to that with the first injections [7]. Patients must be made aware of the fact that there is a risk that they may need to aid bladder emptying by performing clean intermittent self catheterization (CISC) post treatment. Importantly, contraindications include myaesthenia gravis, pregnancy, and, use of gentamicin antibiotic.

Although as yet unlicensed, botulinum toxin type A is now emerging as the preferred second-line treatment (if ACh medication fails) in OAB, and is increasingly being adopted by many urology, neurology, and rehabilitation centers worldwide [7].

Transdermal Oxybutynin Patch

Oxybutynin administered orally is metabolized primarily by the cytochrome P450 enzyme, and metabolites include phenylcyclohexylglycolic acid, which is pharmacologically inactive, and N-desethyloxybutynin (N-DEO), which is pharmacologically active. The active metabolite, N-DEO, has pharmacological effects on the human bladder that is similar to that of oxybutynin observed during in vitro studies. However, it is usually responsible for the majority of side effects associated with anti-muscarinic medication, which prevents the long-term compliance with medication. A trans-dermal continuous controlled delivery device which bypasses the first-pass gastrointestinal and hepatic metabolism, increasing the bioavailability of the active drug, has been introduced. This provides for a greater and more consistent control of absorption into the circulation and the resulting controlled absorption during trans-dermal therapy allows for administration of lower doses, still resulting in therapeutic blood levels, in turn reducing the incidence of dose-related side effects.

In a study comparing the efficacy and safety of the transdermal patch with that of long-acting tolterodine (4 mg) and placebo in previously treated patients, Kentera was found to be an effective and comparable treatment for these patients. However, application site reaction was 23.1% with the Kentera patch [8]. More recently, preliminary findings from the Multicenter Assessment of Transdermal Therapy in OAB with Oxybutynin (MATRIX) study, suggest that open-label Kentera patch produces sustained improvements in OAB symptoms [9] and in the overall quality of life [10], which may be of significant relevance to patients in clinical practice.

Intravaginal Estrogens

Intravaginal estrogens are recommended for the treatment of OAB symptoms in postmenopausal women with vaginal atrophy [1].

Medical Management of Stress Incontinence

Disappointingly, the medical management of stress incontinence is not usually very effective. The only agent with published data is duloxetine, which is a combined norepinephrine and serotonin reuptake inhibitor. In animal models, it has been shown to significantly increase sphincter muscle activity in the storage phase of the micturition cycle. Duloxetine of 80 mg daily, with or without pelvic floor muscle training (PFMT) was compared with PFMT and with no active treatment (sham PFMT and placebo drug) in 201 women with SUI. Significantly, greater reductions in leakage episodes were reported with duloxetine (with or without PFMT), when compared with PFMT alone after 3 months' treatment. Global improvement and quality of life scores indicated greater improvement with duloxetine plus PFMT, when compared with no active treatment. Discontinuation and adverse effect rates (nausea, dizziness, dry mouth, constipation, insomnia, somnolence, asthenia) were significantly higher in duloxetine-treated groups when compared with PFMT or no combined active treatment [11].

In summary, duloxetine is not recommended as a first-line treatment for women with predominant SUI, although it may be offered as a second-line therapy if women prefer pharmacological to surgical treatment or are not suitable for surgical treatment. In clinical practice, if duloxetine is prescribed, women should be counseled about its adverse effects, very carefully.

How to Choose Medical Therapies in OAB and UUI

Management of OAB and UUI should commence with the conservative options discussed initially. Subsequently, if there is no improvement, medical treatments, usually in the form of ACh drugs, can be instituted, either alone or in some cases in combination with bladder training programs. This combination has been shown to result in greater reduction in frequency, but may not necessarily lead to further improvements in incontinence episodes [1]. If first-line medical therapies fail, second-line treatment should be considered. This may be an alternative ACh oral medication, or a transdermal ACh patch. Failure of second-line treatment is an indication for specialist referral for consideration of other diagnoses, or consideration of intravesical BTX-A. Invasive surgical therapies are reserved for the very small minority of patients who fail first- and second-line therapies.

In clinical practice, having excluded any potential contraindications to ACh therapy, the choice of treatment is tailored according to the patient, taking into account, tolerability, potential side effects, convenience of administration, efficacy, and cost [4]. The long-acting (ER or extended life – XL) formulation of these medications can be advantageous, as patients only need to take the tablet once a day to provide a 24-h cover for symptoms. Generally, the more selective agents are much better tolerated. Furthermore, quaternary amine ACh drugs, such as Trospium and Darifenacin, do not cross the blood–brain barrier and thus, are less likely to cause cognitive side effects. This may be of benefit in elderly patients and those with neurological dysfunction. Hence, one treatment is not necessarily appropriate for all patients. Interestingly, according to NICE guidelines, generic oxybutynin should be tried as first-line therapy, but it must be borne in mind that this recommendation was probably based on cost effectiveness, over other factors.

As stated previously, medical management of stress incontinence is not usually very effective. With mixed incontinence, the management is dictated by the form of incontinence that is the dominant one, and this one should be treated first. It is important to counsel these patients that the lesser form of incontinence may remain and be troublesome.

Key Points

1. Urinary incontinence is an extremely prevalent condition and many patients fail to seek medical advice, primarily due to embarrassment.
2. Correct assessment aims primarily to exclude any underlying medical condition that may be causing the incontinence, to establish if it is stress, urge, or mixed incontinence, and to determine the most distressing symptom and its effect on quality of life.
3. First-line medical therapy involves the use of anticholinergic (ACh) medication (also called antimuscarinic), which has been shown to be safe and efficacious in randomized controlled trials against placebo.

4. The introduction of intradetrusor BTX-A injections has allowed the successful second-line therapy of many severely affected cases, not responding to oral first-line treatments.
5. Invasive surgical therapies are reserved for the very small minority of patients who fail first- and second-line medical therapy.

References

1. http://www.nice.org.uk/CG40
2. Herbison P, Hay-Smith J, Ellis G, Moore K (2003) Effectiveness of anticholinergic drugs compared with placebo in the treatment of overactive bladder: systematic review. BMJ 326(7394): 841–844
3. Chapple C, Khullar V, Gabriel Z, Dooley JA (2005) The effects of antimuscarinic treatments in overactive bladder: a systematic review and meta-analysis. Eur Urol 48(1):5–26
4. Chapple C, Khullar V, Gabriel Z, Muston D, Bitoun C, Weinstein D (2008) The effects of antimuscarinic treatments in overactive bladder: an update of a systematic review and meta-analysis. Eur Urol 54(3):543–562
5. Chapple CR, Martinez-Garcia R, Selvaggi L, Toozs-Hobson P, Warnack W, Drogendijk T, Wright DM, Bolodeoku J (2005) for the STAR study group. a comparison of the efficacy and tolerability of solifenacin succinate and extended release tolterodine at treating overactive bladder syndrome: results of the STAR trial. Eur Urol 48(3):464–470
6. Schurch B, de Sèze M, Denys P, Chartier-Kastler E, Haab F, Everaert K, Plante P, Perrouin-Verbe B, Kumar C, Fraczek S, Brin MF (2005) Botox detrusor hyperreflexia study team. botulinum toxin type A is a safe and effective treatment for neurogenic urinary incontinence: results of a single treatment, randomized, placebo controlled 6-month study. J Urol 174(1):196–200
7. Ahmed HU, Shergill IS, Arya M, Shah PJ (2006) Management of detrusor-external sphincter dyssynergia. Nat Clin Pract Urol 3(7):368–380
8. Dmochowski RR, Sand PK, Zinner NR et al (2003) Comparative efficacy and safety of transdermal oxybutynin and oral tolterodine versus placebo in previously treated patients with urge and mixed urinary incontinence. Urology 62:237–242

9. Davila GW, Sand PK, Gonick CW, Parker RL, Dahl NV (2006) Impact of transdermal oxybutynin on nocturia and related symptoms in overactive bladder: results from the MATRIX study. Obstet Gynecol 107:S76

10. Lucente VR, Goldberg RP, Davila GW, Gonick CW, Parker RL, Dahl NV (2006) Impact of transdermal oxybutynin on quality of life in patients with overactive bladder: results from the MATRIX study. Obstet Gynecol 107:176

11. Ghoniem GM, Van Leeuwen JS, Elser DM et al (2005) A randomized controlled trial of duloxetine alone, pelvic floor muscle training alone, combined treatment and no active treatment in women with stress urinary incontinence. J Urol 173(5):1647–1653

Chapter 8
Urinary Tract Infections

Magnus J. Grabe

Introduction

Definitions and Terminology

The definitions and terminology are important clinically, as well as microbiologically, and should be understood before medical treatment is initiated.

Urinary tract infection (UTI) is defined as an inflammatory response of the urothelium to microorganism (usually bacteria) invasion. The presence of bacteria in the urine, as confirmed by culture, is defined as bacteriuria. Bacteriuria may be accompanied by, or occur in the absence of symptoms. The presence of both bacteria and symptoms is therefore, defined as a symptomatic UTI, while the absence of symptoms denotes an asymptomatic bacteriuria (ABU). Practically, UTIs can be classified as complicated (cUTI) and uncomplicated (uUTI). cUTI occurs in the presence of an anatomical or functional abnormality of the urinary tract, or in the presence of an underlying disease that is known to increase the risk of acquiring infection, or failing therapy (Table 8.1). uUTI includes conditions such as cystitis and uncomplicated pyelonephritis. UTI can be isolated/sporadic, recurrent or unresolved. Isolated/

M.J. Grabe (✉)
Department of Urology, Malmö University Hospital, Malmö, Sweden

I.S. Shergill et al. (eds.), *Medical Therapy in Urology*,
DOI 10.1007/978-1-84882-704-2_8,
© Springer-Verlag London Limited 2010

TABLE 8.1.   Main factors associated with a complicated urinary tract infection (UTI).

Associated factor	Examples
Congenital anatomic abnormality	Duplex kidney
	PUJ obstruction
Obstruction of the urinary tract	Reflux
	Stone
	Tumor
	Bladder outlet obstruction
	Extrinsic compressive mass
Neurological dysfunction	Spinal cord injury
	Multiple sclerosis
Concomitant medical disease	Diabetes mellitus
	Immunosuppression

sporadic UTI refers to a >6 month time period between UTIs. Recurrent infections are defined as 3 UTI in 1 year or 2 in 6 months or more. They may be persistent/relapsed or reinfection. Persistent/relapsed means infection with the same bacteria, usually originating from a focus in the urinary tract. This may be secondary to struvite kidney stones, a foreign body, fistula, or chronic bacterial prostatitis. Reinfection refers to infection with different bacteria and is usually due to poor hygiene or UTI related to sexual intercourse. Finally, unresolved UTI implies inadequate treatment because of resistance, infection by different organisms, or a rapid reinfection.

Risk Factors for UTI

A wide range of factors have been identified that can increase susceptibility to UTI, including:

1. *Genetic factors*: nonsecretory status and ABO blood-group antigens.
2. *Biologic factors*: congenital abnormalities, urinary obstruction, prior history of UTI, diabetes, and incontinence or other dysfunction of the urinary tract.
3. *Behavioral*: sexual intercourse and the use of contraceptive devices such as diaphragms, condoms, and spermicides.

4. Urological surgery.
5. *Others*: estrogen deficiency in aging women, previous use of antibiotics.

Epidemiology

UTIs are among the most frequent infections encountered in medical practice. Catheter-associated infections account for approximately 30–40% of healthcare-associated infections, and are an important source of severe UTIs and septicemia. Prevalence studies have shown that up to 10% of patients in urological wards have healthcare-associated complicated infections.

The overall prevalence of bacteriuria in the population is estimated to be 3.5%. Bacteriuria is present in schoolgirls (1–2%) and young women (1–5%). The rate increases with age, and it is estimated that about 25% of all women over the age of 65 years living in their homes, have bacteriuria. One-third of all women are likely to have UTI before the age of 24 years. UTI in men are uncommon until the age of 50 years, when increasing bladder outlet obstruction develops and markedly changes the probability of having UTI. On the other hand, adult men are sensitive to bacterial prostatitis. All patients with indwelling catheters or other long-term urinary tract stents have bacteriuria.

Uropathogens

Clearly, it is of vital importance to know the likely causative pathogens, as this allows the use of appropriate antibiotic treatment. Most UTI are caused by the microorganisms listed in Table 8.2. *Escherichia coli* is the most frequently encountered microbe, present in as many as 75–80% of the community-acquired uUTI and approximately 30–50% of the cUTI. Other main gram negative bacterial species are *Klebsiella* and *Proteus* sp., *Pseudomonas* sp., and gram positive strains such as *Enterococcus faecalis* and some *Staphylococci* species, i.e., *Staphylococcus epidermidis*, *Staphylococcus aureus*, and *Staphylococcus*

TABLE 8.2.   Classification of UTI, causative pathogens and treatment recommendation.

Type of UTI	Bacteria	Antibiotics	Length of treatment (days)	Comments
uUTI (sporadic) cystitis	E. coli (70–80%) Proteus spp. (<5%) Klebsiella spp. (<5%) S. saprophyticus (5–10%) Enterococcus spp. (<5%)	Trimethoprim (± sulphamethox-azole) Nitrofurantoin Second generation cephalosporins	3–5	Avoid flouroquino-lones
uUTI (recurrent)	E. coli (70–80%) Proteus spp. (<5%) Klebsiella spp. (<5%) S. saprophyticus (5–10%) Enterococcus spp. (<5%)	Trimethoprim (± sulphamethox-azole) Nitrofurantoin Second generation cephalosporins Flouroquinolones	7–10	
uUTI (Pyelone-phritis)	E. coli (70–80%) Proteus spp. Klebsiella spp.	Third generation cephalosporins Flouroquinolones Trimethoprim (± sulphamethox-azole)	7–14	
UTI in pregnancy	E. coli (70–80%) Proteus spp. Klebsiella spp.	Refer to local recommendations	7–10	Will require long-term prophylaxis

cUTI	*E. coli* (30–35%) *Proteus, Klebsiella,* and other *Enterobacteriacae spp.* (15–25%) *Pseudomonas* (5–15%) *Enterococcus* (10–20%)	Third generation cephalosporins Flouroquinolones Trimethoprim (± sulphamethoxazole) Aminoglycosides	10–14	Initially, empirical treatment. Then, adjust according to culture result
Septicemia	*E. coli* (30–35%) *Proteus, Klebsiella,* and other *Enterobacteriacae spp.* (15–25%) *Pseudomonas* (5–15%) *Enterococcus* (10–20%)	Third generation cephalosporins Flouroquinolones Trimethoprim (± sulphamethoxazole) Aminoglycosides	10–14	May need dual or triple antibiotic therapy and general supportive treatment
Catheter associated UTI	*E. coli* *Proteus, Klebsiella, Pseudomonas spp.* *Enterococcus faecalis spp.*	According to culture	5–10	No antibiotics in ABU

uUTI uncomplicated urinary tract infection; *cUTI* complicated urinary tract infection; *spp.* species; *ABU* asymptomatic bacteriuria *saprophyticus*, the latter only in female UTI. New microbial profiles and marked changes in susceptibility patterns challenge traditional view on the management of UTI. *Bacillus tuberculosis* can cause progressive destruction of the urinary tract, and it should be noted that Tuberculosis is still a worldwide infectious disease of major importance. Also, the blood fluke *Schistosoma heamatobium* (bilharzias, snail fever) is endemic in defined geographic areas, producing fibrotic lesions, strictures and scars of the ureter and bladder, as well as being a possible underlying cause of bladder cancer.

Diagnosis

The diagnosis of a UTI is based on the combination of symptoms and laboratory findings. Dysuria, urgency, frequency, and suprapubic tenderness characterize lower urinary tract involvement, while fever, flank pain, chills, and shivering usually accompany febrile upper UTI and pyelonephritis. Whilst urine analysis (dipstick test) for leukocytes esterase and nitrate is basic, easy, and reliable in most infections, the gold standard for diagnosis is microscopy, culture, and sensitivity testing of an appropriately collected urine specimen. Bacterial count in terms of colony forming units (cfu) is a very important defining factor for a UTI. For sporadic cystitis in women, a bacterial count of $\geq 10^3$ cfu/mL is accepted, while $\geq 10^4$ cfu/mL is necessary to define an uncomplicated pyelonephritis. A cUTI requires the same symptoms, and $\geq 10^4$ cfu/mL in females and $\geq 10^5$ cfu/mL in males. A urine culture is followed by a susceptibility test that will guide the choice of antibiotics. ABU is defined as the presence of $\geq 10^5$ cfu/mL in at least two consecutive cultures. In case of high fever, chills, and clinical suspicion of severe upper UTI and/or septicemia, it is essential to collect at least two samples of blood for blood culture.

Medical Therapies in Urinary Tract Infections

For daily clinical practical purposes, the aims of the management of UTI are:

1. Effective therapeutic response
2. Prevention of recurrence
3. Reduce the development of resistance of bacterial strains

A detailed review of the literature, amounting to over a 100 pages, is available from the European Association of Urology guidelines, and indeed recommendations for antibiotic treatment are given in these guidelines. For day-to-day practice, the management principles of each type of UTI are discussed presently and the most commonly used antibiotics are reviewed in Table 8.3.

Uncomplicated UTI

Cystitis is the most common uUTI involving only the lower urinary tract, and is seen in both pre- and postmenopausal women. Empiric treatment can be initiated on the basis of symptoms without any further work-up. A short treatment of 3–5 days is sufficient (Table 8.3), due to increased compliance, low cost, and lower risk of adverse side effects. If therapy fails, laboratory testing should be undertaken. A more thorough diagnostic evaluation is indicated for women with evidence of uncomplicated pyelonephritis. This includes a urine analysis, urine culture, and susceptibility testing, and when considered as necessary, radiological evaluation. Involving the renal parenchyma, this infection is more serious and requires a 7–14 days' course of treatment.

UTI in Pregnancy

The consequences of UTI or untreated ABU during pregnancy can be significant, including an increased risk of pyelonephritis, premature delivery, fetal mortality, and pregnancy-induced hypertension. Therefore, screening for bacteriuria is highly recommended. Owing to the importance of UTI in pregnancy, all infections should be adequately treated, usually for 7 days. In addition, it is generally recommended to give long-term prophylaxis in cases of ABU, with low-dose cephalosporin or nitrofurantoin. In cases of acute

TABLE 8.3.   Medical therapy of UTIs.

Name	Mode of action	Dose (adults)	Main adverse effects	Important interactions and contraindications
Trimethoprim	Disrupts folic acid metabolism	200 mg PO BD for treatment 100 mg PO OD for prophylaxis	GI disturbances Allergic reactions (skin rash)	Avoid if known hypersensitivity to trimethoprim Renal insufficiency Avoid during first term of pregnancy Might interact with some contraceptive drugs, cyclosporine and glibencamide
Trimethoprim + sulphamethoxazole	Disrupts folic acid metabolism	160/800 mg × 2 Reduce dose according to renal function	GI disturbances Allergic reactions (skin rash) Renal function reduction	Known hypersensitivity to trimethoprim and/or sulphametoxazol Renal insufficiency Avoid during pregnancy Might interact with some contraceptive drugs, cyclosporine and glibencamide
Mecillinam Piv-mecillinam	Bacterial cell wall synthesis	200 mg × 3 or 400 mg × 2	GI disturbances Allergic reaction (immediate or delayed)	Known hypersensitivity to beta-lactam antibiotics Interaction with probenicid Avoid during last month of pregnancy
Ampicillin + BLI	Bacterial cell wall synthesis	500–750 mg × 2	GI disturbances Allergic reaction (immediate or delayed)	Known hypersensitivity to beta-lactam antibiotics Interaction with probenicid Avoid during last month of pregnancy

Cephalosporins	Bacterial cell wall synthesis	Depends on compound, with dose adapted to clinical severity	GI disturbances (immediate and delayed)	Risk for cross allergic reaction in known hypersensitivity to other beta-lactam antibiotics
Cefotaxime (i.v.) Cefadroxile (oral)		1 g × 3 (iv) 500 mg–1 g × 2		Interaction with probenicid
Nitrofurantoin	30S-inhibitor	100 mg PO QDS for treatment	GI disturbances Fever, headache, muscular pain Pulmonary lesion Leucopenia, anemia	Known glucose-6-phosphodehydrogenas deficiency
		50 mg PO OD for prophylaxis		Directly prior to delivery Metoclopramide
Fosfomycin	Bacterial cell wall synthesis	3 g single dose	GI disturbances	
Flouoroquinolones	DNA gyrase/ topoisomerase	Ciprofloxacin 250–500 mg × 2 Ofloxacin 200–400 mg × 2 Dose adapted to clinical severity Avoid in simple infections	GI disturbances Allergic reactions Headache Secondary infections	Hypersensitivity to flouroquinolones Interaction with tizanidin, antacidum, dairy products, warfarin, etc. History of quinolone-associated tendinitis Dose reduction related to renal function Only on strict indication during pregnancy

TABLE 8.3. (continued)

Name	Mode of action	Dose (adults)	Main adverse effects	Important interactions and contraindications
Aminoglycosides	30S-inhibitors	Gentamicin 3–5 mg/kg/day	Nephrotoxicity Ototoxicity Vestibular toxicity	Caution if reduced renal function Check therapeutic levels

All antibiotics can induce hypersensitive reactions of immediate or delayed type, gastrointestinal side effects such as diarrhea, nausea, vomiting, and hematological disorders such as leucopoenia

All antibiotics can induce a secondary infection. The most common are gastrointestinal infection with *Clostridium difficile*, particularly with cephalosporins, and fungal infection (i.e., *Candida albicans* infection)

pyelonephritis, second or third generation cephalosporins, an aminoglycoside, or an aminopenicillin plus a Beta lactamase inhibitor may be recommended. Importantly, because of adverse effects on fetal development, quinolones, teratcyclines, and trimethoprim are contraindicated in the first trimester of pregnancy. Similarly, sulfonamides should never be used in the final trimester.

Recurrent UTI

As stated previously, recurrent UTI is defined as more than three infections within a year, or 2 UTI in a 6-month period. Recurrent UTIs due to re-infection with different organisms (see definitions above) are common in healthy young women, although they have a structurally and functionally normal urinary tract. Recurrent UTI are seen in women with a family history of UTI and limited intake of fluids and few voiding occasions. Sexual intercourse may increase the frequency of UTI. In elderly women, prolapse, constipation, and concomitant diseases such as diabetes and steroid therapy are the underlying causes for recurrent UTI. UTIs in women are thought to represent ascending infections, with bacteria colonizing the perineum and ascending the short female urethra with ease, causing a symptomatic UTI. It is because of this mechanism that sexual intercourse is thought to play a role, with sexual activity causing bacteria from the vagina to be introduced through the urethra into the bladder.

The medical management is based on the use of antibiotics as treatment and/or prophylaxis. Antibiotic prophylaxis reduces the number of episodes, but is controversial in view of the development of antibiotic resistance. Short courses "on demand" is an alternative strategy – this is also referred to as "patient-initiated" or "self-start" therapy. Furthermore, post intercourse prophylaxis is recommended in those women whose UTI are associated with sexual intercourse.

In addition, a combination of simple measures also seems to reduce the rate of UTIs. This includes a high intake of fluids, regular urination (in order to avoid distension of the bladder and residual urine with bacterial growth opportunities), voiding postintercourse, and avoidance of spermicides (which may enhance *E. coli* adherence to urothelial cells through reducing natural vaginal flora).

Newer investigational alternative prophylactic methods include immunotherapy (including vaccination with bacterial extracts), probiotic treatment, and cranberry extracts (Vaccinium Macrocarpon). Ingestion of bioyoghurt is thought to increase commensal lactobacilli in the vaginal flora, creating an acidic environment and thus, hindering bacterial colonization of the vagina, which is thought to precede urethral and bladder involvement. Cranberry juice has been shown to decrease symptomatic recurrences of UTIs by prevention of *E. Coli* adherence to the urothelium.

With persistent/relapsed UTI, multiple infections with the same organism suggest pathology within the urinary tract. This group needs focused investigations to elucidate the cause, which is then managed appropriately.

Asymptomatic UTI

It is recommended not to treat ABU, except during pregnancy. Only patients exhibiting episodes of symptomatic bacteriuria should be given antibiotics. The same recommendations as for uUTI are valid.

Complicated UTI

cUTI requires imaging investigation for underlying cause and risk-factor assessment. The treatment is medical and/or surgical correction of the underlying causative factor. A urine culture and blood culture is highly recommended. Initially, the medical treatment is empirical and initiated with at least one, but usually two, intravenous antibiotics for 1–3 days, until the fever is controlled, and the laboratory findings show a stabilization or decrease of the inflammatory process (Table 8.2 and Fig. 8.1). Subsequently, urine cultures can guide in the choice of antibiotics, and careful monitoring with additional supportive measures, has to be undertaken.

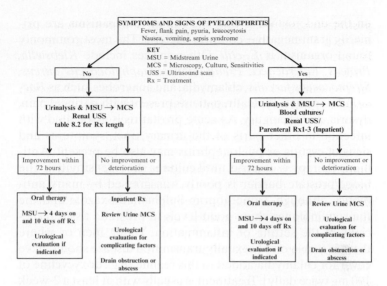

FIGURE 8.1. Simplified algorithm for investigation and treatment of UTI.

Septicemia

Sepsis is a serious life-threatening condition requiring aggressive and intensive antibiotic treatment similar to that of cUTI. Urine and blood cultures are imperative. Monitoring and full life-support treatment, with the involvement of anesthetic/intensivist colleagues, is mandatory. Initial treatment with two antibiotics is recommended (Table 8.2). It must be remembered that even with this aggressive and intense approach, morbidity and mortality remains very high.

Acute Prostatitis

Acute bacterial prostatitis is considered as a subtype of UTI and is thought to arise either as a result of reflux of infected urine into the glandular prostatic tissue via the prostatic and ejaculatory ducts, or from ascending urethral (sexual) infection from the meatus. The use of antibiotic treatment is based on the understanding that the causative organisms are primarily gram-negative, coliform bacteria. The most commonly found organism is *E. coli*. Other species include *Klebsiella*, *Proteus*, *Enterococci*, *Pseudomonas*, *Staphylococcus aureus*, *Streptococcus faecalis*, chlamydia, and anaerobes such as *Bacteriodes* species. Typically, patients present with perineal pain, dysuria, and strangury. As acute prostatitis is associated with infection in other parts of the urinary tract, symptoms and signs of cystitis or pyelonephritis may also be present. Antibiotic therapy is empiric, until cultures show sensitivities. The blood/prostate barrier is poorly transgressed by many antibiotics, although Trimethoprim-Sulphamethoxazole and the fluoroquinolones show good levels in prostatic tissue, especially in the setting of inflammation. Young men or where there is suspicion of sexually-transmitted disease should have cover for chlamydia added to this regime (e.g., doxycycline of 100 mg twice daily). Treatment is usually with at least a 2-week course, and occasionally may continue for up to 6–8 weeks. If there is a lack of response to medical treatment, imaging is indicated. If the complication of prostatic abscess has developed, surgical drainage is indicated.

Healthcare-Associated Infections

Global prevalence studies have shown that healthcare-associated infections are common in urology, amounting to some 10–14% of patients in urological ward. The largest group is ABU, cystitis, pyelonephritis, and sepsis. The main underlying causes or risk factors are treatment with an indwelling catheter, nephrostomy tube or JJ-stent, obstruction of the urinary tract, stone disease, recent antibiotic treatment, and recent hospitalization.

Reduce Resistance Development

There is a general trend toward increased resistance of bacteria to standard antimicrobial agents. This is explained by the overuse and misuse of antibiotics and has to be combated by a judicious and evidence-based use of antimicrobial agents.

Key Points

1. UTI are among the most frequent uncomplicated infections in the community. Indwelling catheters are the underlying cause of most of the healthcare-associated UTI, usually complicated and often severe.
2. Urine culture is a key diagnostic procedure. The result is obtained after the initiation of empiric treatment, and leads to relevant adjustment according to the needs.
3. Sporadic cystitis requires only a short 2–5 day treatment, while an ascending pyelonephritis needs a 7–14 day antibiotic treatment.
4. Severe complicated UTI and sepsis can be life-threatening. Treatment has to be initiated without any delay after primary clinical diagnosis.
5. All antibiotics can give both gastrointestinal disturbances and allergic reactions. Knowledge about the renal function is important. Initial treatment can usually be started with normal dosage, but the following doses must be adjusted to the renal function and the patients' general condition.

Further Reading

1. Grabe M, Bishop MC, Bjerklund Johansen TE, Botto H et al. Urological infections. Guidelines of the European Association of Urology. EAU Guidelines Office (publ). March 2009, pp 1–109. ISBN-13:978-90-70244-88-0. http://www.uroweb. com
2. Ahmed H, Silhi N, Tsiouris A, Emberton M (2007) Urinary tract infection. In: Shergill IS, Arya M, Patel HR, Gill IS (eds) Urological emergencies in hospital medicine. Quay Books, London, pp 103–116
3. Bjerklund-Johansen T, Cek M, Naber K, Stratchounski L et al (2007) Prevalence of hospital-acquired urinary tract infections in urology departments. Eur Urol 51:1100–1112
4. Naber K, Schito G, Botto H, Palou J, Mazzei T (2008) Surveillance study in europe and brazil on clinical aspects and antimicrobial resistance epidemiology in females with cystitis

(ARESC): implications for empiric therapy. Eur Urol 54: 1164–1178

5. Stamm WE (2002) Scientific and clinical challenges in the management of urinary tract infections. Am J Med 113(1A): 1S–4S

Chapter 9
Bladder Pain Syndrome/ Interstitial Cystitis

Paul Irwin

Introduction

Bladder pain syndrome (BPS) should be regarded as a true pain syndrome (a collection of symptoms and signs which, together, characterize a particular condition or disease) rather than an end-organ disease. The term "interstitial cystitis" (IC) has been a misleading name for a condition in which true bladder inflammation is seen only in a small subset of patients with chronic bladder pain. Furthermore, the lack of consensus as to what constitutes IC has hindered progress in the understanding of what is now called BPS. By definition, BPS/IC it consists of "the complaint of suprapubic pain related to bladder filling accompanied by other symptoms, such as increased daytime and nighttime frequency, in the absence of proven urinary infection or other obvious pathology" [1, 2]. The precise etiology and pathogenesis of BPS/IC is unknown, but the overwhelming majority of patients with BPS/IC are female (F:M = 10:1).

The syndrome has many hallmarks of a chronic inflammatory disease, but its clinical presentation and course are analogous to Chronic Regional Pain Syndrome (formerly known as Reflex Sympathetic Dystrophy) [3]. The inflammatory features of BPS/IC are believed to be secondary, probably induced by the leakage of urine or toxic solutes through the urothelium.

P. Irwin (✉)
Michael Heal Department of Urology, Mid-Cheshire Hospitals NHS Foundation Trust Leighton Hospital, Crewe, UK
e-mail: paul.irwin@mcht.nhs.uk

I.S. Shergill et al. (eds.), *Medical Therapy in Urology*,
DOI 10.1007/978-1-84882-704-2_9,
© Springer-Verlag London Limited 2010

However, whether this is a result of a defect in the protective glycosoaminoglycans (GAG) layer or not is unclear. While minor qualitative defects have been identified in the composition of the GAG layer, there is no evidence of any quantitative defect. The inflammatory features consist of perineural and perivascular infiltration of lymphocytes, plasma cells, neutrophils, and mast cells. None of these features is unique to BPS/IC. There is evidence that patients with BPS/IC have ischemic bladders, probably as a result of a neurovascular mechanism [4, 5]. Impaired bladder perfusion might account for a functional defect in the urothelial barrier. Neurobiological features of BPS/IC include a neoprofileration of nerve fibers in the suburothelium and derusor, upregulation of afferent C-fibers which take on the properties of Aδ fibers (with a lower firing threshold and more tonic firing), and the enhancement of sodium, calcium, and TRPV1 pain channels [6].

In summary, the precise etiology and pathogenesis of BS/IC is unknown.

Clinical Assessment

The diagnosis must always be questioned, especially when the patient fails to respond to treatment. All common causes of pelvic pain and frequency must be excluded on an active and ongoing basis [2, 7]. These may include filling and voiding cystometry if bladder outlet obstruction or detrusor overactivity is suspected, although the latter may coexist with BPS/IC. Cystoscopy under general anesthetic is not mandatory, but may be performed to exclude bladder cancer or carcinoma in situ and to classify the condition [1, 2]. The potassium sensitivity test is no longer felt to have any indication in diagnosis. A suggested mode of assessment and investigation is shown in the flow diagram (Fig. 9.1), and is based on European Association of Urology (EAU) guidelines.

Overview of Management

BPS/IC can be a very frustrating condition to manage, both for patients and their clinicians. Importantly, it cannot be managed single-handedly. Patients must be assured that they

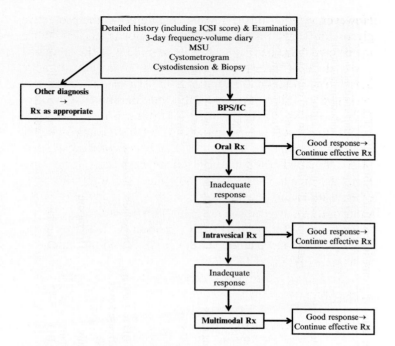

FIGURE 9.1.   Management algorithm for BPS/IC based on EAU guidelines.

can obtain advice and help at short notice, so an empathic team of nurses and pain management specialists is essential. All patients should join a support group. Dietary and behavioral modifications may help in some cases.

Treatment is aimed at symptomatic relief rather than cure, and multimodal treatment is recommended [8, 9]. Commonly-used agents are shown in Table 9.1 It is also advisable to make the patient aware at an early stage that surgery may be an option if conservative strategies fail.

Medical Therapies in BPS/IC

As the exact etiology and pathophysiology of BPS/IC remains unknown, one of the most challenging problems, in terms of assessing treatment options from the many published clinical

TABLE 9.1. Medical therapy of bladder pain syndrome/interstitial cystitis (BPS/IC).

Name	Mode of action	Dose	Main side effects	Important interactions and contraindications
Pentosan polysulfate (PPS)	Replenishment of glycosoaminoglycans (GAG) layer Possible free-radical scavenger	100 mg tds	Hypersensitivity, allopecia, diarrhea	Caution with those on oral anticoagulants, hemorrhage and thrombocytopenia
Hydroxyzine	Mast cell stabilizer Antihistamine Hypnotic	25 mg nocte	Dry mouth, drowsiness	Potentiates effects of CNS depressants
Amitriptyline	Central + peripheral anticholinergic action Inhibits re-uptake of serotonin + noradrenaline Sedative	10–50 mg daily	Dry mouth, drowsiness	Caution with monoamine oxidase inhibitors and anticholinergics
Gabapentin	Central pain control Inhibition of micturition reflex	300 mg BD to 1,800 mg daily increased over 2 weeks	Drowsiness, dizziness	
Tolterodine XL	Antimuscarinic agent	4 mg daily	Dry mouth	
Solifenacin		10 mg daily		
Cimetidine	Antihistamine	300 mg BD	Diarrhea	Caution with those on warfarin

Dimethyl sulphoxide (DMSO)	Antiinflammatory Free-radical scavenger Local anesthetic Carrier for other agents	50 mL 50% solution 2-weekly over 3 months	Temporary flare-up of symptoms Garlic odor	
Hyaluronic acid	GAG replacement	40 mg once weekly for 6–8 weeks	Bruising, redness, swelling	
Intravesical lidocaine	Pain relief, especially for bad flare-ups or following cystoscopy/ cystodistension	10 mL of 2% lidocaine followed by 10 mL of 8.4% Na bicarbonate	None	
Lumbar epidural bupivicaine infusion	Pain relief, especially for bad flare-ups or following cystoscopy/ cystodistension	As per local guidelines	Hypotension	Caution in those on anticoagulants

trials, is the lack of harmony between studies in terms of inclusion and exclusion criteria. A brief review of the commonly used agents is presented now, followed by an algorithm of recommended medical management of patients with BPS/IC.

Pentosan Polysulfate (PPS) – Elmiron

PPS is thought to substitute for a defect in the GAG layer and has been evaluated in double-blind, placebo-controlled studies [2]. Subjective improvement of pain, urgency, frequency, but not nocturia, was reported in patients taking the drug when compared with placebo. In addition, in an open multicentre study, PPS had a more favorable effect in classic IC disease [10]. In contrast, a prospective randomized controlled trial (RCT) Comparing PPS and hydroxine against placebo failed to demonstrate a statistically significant outcome for either drug, though PPS approached statistical significance ($p = 0.064$) [11]. Combination therapy showed the highest response rate of 40% when compared to 13% with placebo. For patients with an initial minor response to PPS, additional subcutaneous administration of heparin appeared helpful [12]. Importantly, only a tiny fraction of oral PPS is absorbed and presented to the bladder urothelium, and treatment must be persisted with over many months before a clinical improvement is obtained. This may affect patient compliance with this medication. Alternatively, intravesical treatment can be considered based on evidence from a double-blind placebo-controlled study on 20 patients, in which four patients in the PPS group and two patients in the placebo group gained significant symptomatic relief [13].

Hyaluronic Acid (Cystistat)

Hyaluronic acid is a natural proteoglycan which can be instilled intravesically with the aim of repairing defects in the GAG layer. A response rate of 56% at week 4 and 71% at week 7 was reported in 25 patients treated with hyaluronic acid [14]. After week 24, effectiveness decreased, but there was no significant toxicity. In a 3-month, prospective, nonrandomized study of 20 patients, followed up for 3 years, the effect of intravesical hyaluronic acid on BPS/IC symptoms was found to be beneficial in approximately half of the patients [15]. In this study, 11 patients chose to continue treatment beyond the initial trial, and modest beneficial long-term effects were noted in about two-thirds of patients. Another study [16] demonstrated a similar favorable effect of hyaluronic acid on pain reduction, with improvements in visual analog pain scores, irrespective of bladder capacity.

Chondroitin Sulfate (Uracyst)

Two nonrandomized, uncontrolled, open-label pilot studies have demonstrated beneficial effects in patients treated with intravesical chondroitin sulfate [2]. In the first study [17], 18 patients were administered with 40 mL instillation intravesically once a week for 4 weeks and then, once a month for 12 months. Thirteen of the 18 patients were followed for the entire 13-month study. Twelve of these patients responded to treatment within 3–12 weeks. A total of 6/13 (46.2%) showed a good response, 2/13 (15.4%) had a fair response, 4/13 (30.8%) had a partial response, and 1/13 (7.7%) showed no response. In the second trial [18], 24 refractory patients with BPS/IC were treated with high-dose chondroitin sulfate instillations twice weekly for 2 weeks, then weekly with 0.2% solution for 4 weeks, and monthly thereafter for 1 year. The average symptom improvement reported in 20 patients completing the trial was 73.1% (range 50–95%). The time to optimum response was 4–6 months. Reasssuringly, phase II/III nonrandomized, uncontrolled community-based open-label efficacy and safety studies are being carried out at present and expected to report shortly.

Dimethyl Sulfoxide (DMSO)

DMSO is a potent organic solvent and water-soluble liquid that penetrates the cell membranes and has anti-inflammatory, local anesthetic collagenolytic and muscle relaxant properties. In addition, DMSO is also a scavenger of the intracellular hydroxyl radical, which is believed to be an important trigger of the inflammatory process. However, despite these features, the clinical evidence for its use in BPS/IC is actually limited. In a controlled crossover trial [19], patients received intravesical instillations of 50% DMSO solution and placebo every 2 weeks for two sessions of four treatments each. Subjective improvement was noted in 53% of patients receiving DMSO vs. 18% receiving placebo, and objective improvement in 93 and 35%, respectively. Other uncontrolled trials with DMSO have reported response rates of 50–70% [20]. After DMSO instillations, a residual treatment effect lasting 16–72 months could be seen [21]. DMSO is contraindicated during urinary tract infections or shortly after bladder biopsy, and it may temporarily cause a garlic-like odor. In summary, although some studies have demonstrated clinical efficacy with DMSO, in clinical practice, this treatment is generally tolerated poorly and in some circumstances, may actually exacerbate the symptoms.

Amitryptiline

Amitriptyline is a tricyclic antidepressant that has both central and peripheral anticholinergic effects. It also has antihistamine and sedative properties. It is best taken at night, and the dose can be self-titrated, beginning with 20 mg and increasing gradually to 100 mg.

Hydroxyzine

A tricyclic antihistamine, has little evidence to support its use, although its sedative effects are useful.

Gabapentin

Gabapentin is widely used in the treatment of neuropathic pain. Although its mode of action is unknown, it is believed to block calcium channels centrally. It may also have an inhibitory effect on the micturition reflex. It is a safe and effective means of long-term pain suppression.

Botulinum Toxin

Intravesical injection of botulinum toxin has shown promising results in two small open-label studies [22, 23], but it is generally accepted that it is difficult to administer this drug in BPS/IC patients because of the small bladder capacity and bleeding at the injection sites.

Analgesics

It would appear to be intuitive that analgesics would be of benefit in BPS/IC, as pain is often a dominant presenting symptom. However, pain relief is disappointing, because the visceral pain experienced in BPS/IC responds poorly to analgesic drugs. Interestingly, no systematic studies have been presented on conventional analgesic medications. Importantly, although short-term opioids may be indicated for breakthrough pain, especially during flare-ups, long-term opioids should only be used in exceptional circumstances and under close surveillance, after all other available treatments have been exhausted so as to avoid the risk of opioid dependency

Other Medical Treatments

Genetic studies have highlighted approximately 1,000 genes that are twice as common in BPS/IC as in normal healthy controls. Many of these up-regulated genes are expressed in leukocytes. However, there is no clear evidence that BPS/IC is a primary immunological entity; like the histological findings (lymphocyte infiltration, monocytes, and mast cells), the immunological findings are generally felt to be secondary features of a condition whose nature remains unclear. Despite this, immunosuppressants, particularly cyclosporin, have been associated with quite remarkable clinical (and cystoscopic) improvements [24]. Empirical antibiotic treatment may also provide symptomatic relief in spite of urine being sterile. Although detrusor overactivity is not a feature of BPS/IC, troublesome urgency and frequency may sometimes be controlled with an anticholinergic agent.

Management Algorithm – Based on EAU Guidelines

Overall, the treatments with the strongest evidence to support their use in BPS/IC are amitriptyline, PPS, and intravesical DMSO [2, 8, 9]. With the evidence base available, it is difficult to make clear-cut recommendations, but based on current clinical practice, it seems that multimodal treatment is recommended in order to obtain *symptom control*, and this combination should be maintained in the long term. A good combination of agents used by the author [7] includes GAG replacement therapy (oral PPS or intravesical hyaluronic acid), amitriptyline, gabapentin, and an anticholinergic agent (tolterodine or solifenacin).

Periodic *"rescue" treatment* may be required for flare-ups. Sometimes, empirical antibiotics are effective despite the urine being sterile. However, a very useful treatment is the instillation of 2% lignocaine (10 mL) followed by 10 mL of 8.5% sodium bicarbonate. This is particularly useful following cystoscopic interventions [25].

Key Points

1. Previously called interstitial cystitis (IC) and Bladder Pain Syndrome (BPS), the complaint of suprapubic pain related to bladder filling, accompanied by other lower urinary tract symptoms is now referred to as BPS/IC and is a diagnosis of exclusion.
2. BPS/IC can be a very frustrating condition to manage, both for patients and their clinicians.
3. The aim of treatment is to alleviate symptoms and is best achieved through an integrated team approach, with the use of multimodal drug treatment, psychological support, and pain management.
4. Several oral and intravesical the rapies have shown to be effective in treating this condition (primarily GAG-replacement therapy), but further large randomized controlled trials are desperately needed to provide a good evidence base.
5. Surgery remains a final option, although it should be discussed early in the course of the patient's management.

References

1. Bade JJ, Laseur M, Nieuwenburg A, van der Weele LT, Mensink HJ (1997) A placebo-controlled study of intravesical pentosanpolysulphate for the treatment of interstitial cystitis. Br J Urol 79(2):168–171

 2. Daha LK, Riedl CR, Lazar D, Hohlbrugger G, Pfluger H
    (2005) Do cystometric findings predict the results of intravesical
    hyaluronic acid in women with interstitial cystitis? Eur Urol
    47(3):393–397; discussion 397
 3. Fall M, Oberpenning F, Peeker R (2008) Treatment of bladder
    pain syndrome/interstitial cystitis 2008; can we make evidence-
    based decisions? Eur Urol 54(1):65–75
 4. Fritjofsson A, Fall M, Juhlin R, Persson BE, Ruutu M (1987)
    Treatment of ulcer and nonulcer interstitial cystitis with so-
    dium pentosanpolysulfate: a multicenter trial. J Urol 138(3):
    508–512
 5. Giannantoni A, Porena M, Costantini E, Zucchi A, Mearini L,
    Mearini E (2008) Botulinum A toxin intravesical injection in pa-
    tients with painful bladder syndrome: 1-year followup. J Urol
    179(3):1031–1034
 6. http://www.uroweb.org/fileadmin/tx_eauguidelines/2009/Full/
    CPP.pdf
 7. Irwin P (2008) Recent developments in BPS/IC. Urol News
    12(10):6–11
 8. Irwin P, Galloway NTM (1993) Impaired bladder perfusion in
    interstitial cystitis: a study using laser doppler flowmetry. J Urol
    149(4):890–892
 9. Irwin P, Samsudin A (2005) Reinvestigation of patients with a
    diagnosis of interstitial cystitis: common things are sometimes
    common. J Urol 174(2):584–587
10. Kanai A, de Groat W, Chai T, Hultgren S, Fowler C, Fry C (2006)
    Symposium on urothelial dysfunction: pathophysiology and
    novel therapies. J Urol 175(5):1624–1629
11. Karsenty G, AlTaweel W, Hajebrahimi S, Corcos J (2006) Effica-
    cy of interstitial cystitis treatments: a review. EAU-EBU Update
    Series 4:47–61
12. Morales A, Emerson L, Nickel JC, Lundie M (1996) Intravesical
    hyaluronic acid in the treatment of refractory interstitial cystitis.
    J Urol 156(1):45–48
13. Nordling J, Jorgensen S, Kallestrup E (2001) Cystistat for the
    treatment of interstitial cystitis: a 3-year followup study. Urology
    57(6 Suppl 1):123
14. Perez-Marrero R, Emerson LE, Feltis JT (1988) A controlled study
    of dimethyl sulfoxide in interstitial cystitis. J Urol 140(1):36–39
15. Pontari MA, Hanno PM, Ruggieri MR (1999) Comparison of
    bladder blood flow in patients with and without interstitial
    cystitis. J Urol 162(2):330–334

16. Ramsay AK, Small DR, Conn IG (2007) Intravesical botulinum toxin type A in chronic interstitial cystitis: results of a pilot study. Surgeon 5(6):331–333

17. Rössberger J, Fall M, Peeker R (2005) Critical appraisal of dimethyl sulfoxide treatment for interstitial cystitis: discomfort, side-effects and treatment outcome. Scand J Urol Nephrol 39(1):73–77

18. Sairanen J, Hotakainen K, Tammela TL, Stenman UH, Ruutu M (2008) Urinary epidermal growth factor and interleukin-6 levels in patients with painful bladder syndrome/interstitial cystitis treated with cyclosporine or pentosan polysulfate sodium. Urology 71(4):630–633

19. GR Sant (ed) (1996) Interstitial cystitis – the neurovascular perspective in interstitial cystitis. Raven Press, New York

20. Sant GR, LaRock DR (1994) Standard intravesical therapies for interstitial cystitis. Urol Clin North Am 21(1):73–83

21. Sant GR, Propert KJ, Hanno PM, Burks D, Culkin D, Diokno AC, Hardy C, Landis JR, Mayer R, Madigan R, Messing EM, Peters K, Theoharides TC, Warren J, Wein AJ, Steers W, Kusek JW, Nyberg LM (2003) Interstitial cystitis clinical trials group. a pilot clinical trial of oral pentosan polysulfate and oral hydroxyzine in patients with interstitial cystitis. J Urol 170(3):810–815

22. Sorensen RB (2003) Chondroitin sulphate in the treatment of interstitial cystitis and chronic inflammatory disease of the urinary bladder. Eur Urol 2:16–18

23. Steinhoff G (2003) The efficacy of chondroitin sulfate in treating interstitial cystitis. Eur Urol 2:14–16

24. van de Merwe JP, Nordling J, Bouchelouche P, Bouchelouche K, Cervigni M, Daha LK, Elneil S, Fall M, Hohlbrugger G, Irwin P, Mortensen S, van Ophoven A, Osborne JL, Peeker R, Richter B, Riedl C, Sairanen J, Tinzl M, Wyndaele JJ (2008) Diagnostic criteria, classification and nomenclature for painful bladder syndrome/interstitial cystitis. Eur Urol 53(1):60–67

25. van Ophoven A, Heinecke A, Hertle L (2005) Safety and efficacy of concurrent application of oral pentosan polysulfate and subcutaneous low-dose heparin for patients with interstitial cystitis. Urology 66(4):707–711

Chapter 10
Chronic Prostatitis/Chronic Pelvic Pain Syndrome

José M. Reyes and Michael A. Pontari

Introduction

CP/CPPS is a poorly understood condition that causes significant morbidity. Affecting 5–12% of men worldwide, it is classified, according to the National Institutes of Health (NIH) classification of prostatitis, as Category III (Table 10.1). CP/CPPS is defined as genitourinary pain in the absence of uropathogenic bacteria, detected by standard microbiologic methods [1]. The symptoms are similar to other forms of prostatitis, including lower urinary tract symptoms accompanied by moderate to severe pain in the genitalia, perineum, suprapubic area, and/or lower back lasting for at least 3 months. Patients may also experience diminished sexual health. Overall, CP/CPPS accounts for approximately 90% of prostatitis cases. The diagnosis of CP/CPPS is that of exclusion, and it is important that in the work-up, no reversible cause of the symptoms is missed. The etiology of CP/CPPS is unknown, although many theories exist.

M.A. Pontari (✉)
Department of Urology, Temple University School of Medicine,
Philadelphia, PA, USA
e-mail: Michel.Pontari@tuhs.temple.edu

I.S. Shergill et al. (eds.), *Medical Therapy in Urology*,
DOI 10.1007/978-1-84882-704-2_10,
© Springer-Verlag London Limited 2010

TABLE 10.1.   National Institutes of Health (NIH) classification of prostatitis [1].

Category	Type	Description
I	Acute bacterial prostatitis	Sudden onset of fever and dysuria Bacterial infection (+) Urine culture
II	Chronic bacterial prostatitis	Dysuria Relapsing episodes of urinary tract infection
III	Chronic prostatitis/Chronic pelvic pain syndrome (CP/CPPS)	
	IIIA inflammatory CP/CPPS	(+) WBCs in semen, EPS, and VB3
	IIIB noninflammatory CP/CPPS	No WBCs in semen, EPS, and VB3
IV	Asymptomatic inflammatory prostatitis	Diagnosed incidentally (Histological)

WBC white blood cells; *EPS* expressed prostatic secretions; *VB3* voided bladder urine-3

Pathophysiology and Anatomy

The term "prostatitis" in CP/CPPS is a bit of a misnomer, as whether or not the prostate is actually the source in men with CP/CPPS has been questioned. In one study, prostatic inflammation was detected in only 33% of men with CP/CPPS who had undergone transperineal prostate biopsy [2]. Disappointingly, the etiology of CP/CPPS is unknown. Theories about the causes of CP/CPPS have focused predominantly on infectious, neurological, psychological, and genetic origins.

As the definition states, uropathogenic bacteria are absent in CP/CPPS. Research comparing prostate tissue from patients with CP/CPPS with those from controls using the polymerase chain reaction (PCR), has shown no difference in the rates of positive findings of bacteria [3]. One theory supporting infection as a cause of CP/CPPS is based on an occult or untreated infection that in susceptible men goes on to cause chronic pain after the acute infection has resolved. In a study of over 30,000 health professionals, men reporting a history of sexually transmitted disease had 1.8-fold greater odds of a self-reported history of prostatitis [4].

Another hypothesis is a dysfunction of the nervous system, which appears to be sound given that CP/CPPS patients suffer pain without a definitive cause. In one study, rat prostate and bladder were chemically irritated causing c-fos expression at spinal cord levels L6 and S1, as well as plasma extravasation at the respective dermatome [5]. These dermatomes correspond with the umbilicus to the mid thigh in humans, which is the common distribution of pain in individuals with CPPS.

In chronic pain syndromes, such as reflex sympathetic dystrophy and fibromyalgia, it has been shown that patients have heightened responses to noxious heat stimuli in areas of chronic pain. In a recent study, men with CPPS, when compared with asymptomatic controls, had heightened responses to noxious heat stimuli provided to the perineum and no difference to the anterior thigh [6].

There is unquestionably a psychological component to CP/CPPS. The important question is whether or not this is a cause or effect of the condition, as the symptoms of CP/CPPS can be psychologically stressful. Psychological stress and depression have been associated with CP/CPPS flare ups, and affect the perception of pain. Although a patient's psyche most definitely affects this condition, one must not attribute a patient's symptoms totally to a psychogenic cause or a pathologic cause may be missed.

Several genetic differences between men with CP/CPPS and controls have been identified, including differences in the DNA sequence or polymorphisms in the promoter regions of several cytokines. The cytokines may function as proinflammatory or inhibitory, and it is the imbalance of the complex network of cytokines that may cause CP/CPPS. Differences have also been reported in the frequency of three alleles near the phosphoglycerate kinase (PGK) gene between CPPS patients and controls, raising the possibility of androgen insensitivity or dysfunction in the pathogenesis of men with CPPS [7].

Assessment

CP/CPPS is a diagnosis of exclusion. In working up a patient with pelvic pain, it is important to rule out a reversible cause of symptoms. There is no standard evaluation method to men with CP/CPPS. However, the following points should be covered in the assessment. Detailed history, including determination of the severity of disease, assessed only by means of a reliable validated symptom-scoring instrument, such as the National Institute of Health chronic prostatitis symptom index (NIH-CPSI). This objective marker is then also useful in monitoring subsequent disease progression and treatment response. Physical examination should include DRE if aged >50 or if prostate cancer is suspected. In patients with pelvic pain and an elevated PSA, a prostate biopsy should be done. Laboratory diagnosis has been classically based on the Stamey four-glass test for bacterial localization [8]. Besides a sterile premassage urine (voided bladder urine-2 [VB2]), CP/CPPS shows less than 10,000 colony-forming units of uropathogenic bacteria in expressed prostatic secretions (EPS) and insignificant numbers of leucocytes or bacterial growth in ejaculate. Uroflowrate and ultrasound with postvoid residual volume will establish the presence of bladder outflow obstruction. Interestingly, formal urodynamic studies in men with CP/CPPS demonstrate decreased urinary flow rates, incomplete relaxation of the bladder neck and prostatic urethra, as well as abnormally high urethral closure pressure at rest. If hematuria, microscopic or gross, is noted during work-up for pelvic pain, then cystoscopy, urine cytology, and upper tract imaging should be obtained.

Medical Therapies in CP/CPPS

When a diagnosis of CP/CPPS is made, the challenge of a proper treatment regimen begins. Unfortunately, as CP/CPPS is a poorly understood condition, the medical treatment

TABLE 10.2.   Medical therapy of CP/CPPS.

Name	Drug class	Mode of action	Oral dosage	Main side effects	Important contraindications and potential interactions
Levofloxacin (Levaquin®)	Fluoroquinolone	Inhibits DNA-gyrase in susceptible organisms, promotes breakage of DNA strands	500 mg daily for 4–6 weeks	Nausea, rash, headache Black box warning: tendonitis and tendon rupture	Contraindications: hypersensitivity to drug class Potential interactions: Alfuzosin – ↑QTc, Coumadin – ↑INR
Ciprofloxacin (Cipro®)	Fluoroquinolone	Inhibits DNA-gyrase in susceptible organisms, promotes breakage of DNA strands	500 mg Q12 h for 4–6 weeks	Nausea, rash, headache Black box warning: tendonitis and tendon rupture	Contraindications: Hypersensitivity to drug Potential interactions: Coumadin – ↑INR
Tamsulosin (Flomax®)	α1a-blocker	Inhibits α1a-receptors in the prostate and bladder neck, causing smooth muscle relaxation and improvement of urine flow (selective α-blockade)	0.4 mg Q HS (can titrate to 0.8 mg Q HS)	Orthostatic hypotension, headache, dizziness, abnormal ejaculation	Contraindications: Hypersensitivity to drug Potential interactions: β-blocker – ↑Orthostatic effects

(continued)

Table 10.2.   (continued)

Name	Drug class	Mode of action	Oral dosage	Main side effects	Important contraindications and potential interactions
Alfuzosin (Uroxatrol®)	α1a-blocker	Inhibits α1a-receptors in the prostate and bladder neck, causing smooth muscle relaxation and improvement of urine flow (selective α-blockade)	10 mg daily	Dizziness, fatigue, headache	Contraindications: Hypersensitivity to drug, Moderate or severe hepatic insufficiency, CYP3A4 inhibitors (e.g., ketoconazole, ritonavir)\n\nPotential interactions: β-blocker – ↑Orthostatic effects, Levofloxacin – ↑QTc
Doxazosin (Cardura®)	α1-blocker	Inhibits α1-receptors causing vasodilation, and relaxation of prostate and bladder neck smooth muscle	Start 1–2 mg daily, titrate to 4–8 mg daily	Orthostatic hypotension, headache, dizziness, weakness	Contraindications: Hypersensitivity to drug\n\nPotential interactions: β-blocker – ↑Orthostatic effects
Ibuprofen (Advil®, Motrin®)	Nonsteroidal anti-inflammatory drugs (NSAIDs)	Decreases the activity of the enzyme cyclooxygenase, inhibiting prostaglandin synthesis	400–800 mg BID-TID	Dizziness, itching, nervousness, abdominal pain/cramps/distress, dyspepsia, tinnitus, ↓platelet function	Contraindications: Hypersensitivity to drug class, Gastrointestinal bleeding

Drug	Class	Mechanism	Dosage	Side effects	Contraindications/Interactions
Nortriptyline (Pamelor®)	Tricyclic Antidepressant	Inhibits presynaptic neuronal membrane reuptake of serotonin and norepinephrine	10 mg QHS, titrate up to 75 mg QHS	Anticholinergic effects, sedation	Contraindications: Hypersensitivity to drug, Use of MAO-I within 14 days, recovery from acute MI. Potential interactions: MAO-I – serotonin syndrome, Alfuzosin – ↑QTc, Coumadin – ↑INR, Ciprofloxacin – ↑QTc
Gabapentin (Neurontin®)	Antiepileptic	Bind to voltage-gate calcium channels, and may modulate the release of excitatory neurotransmitters	100–800 mg TID	Somnolence, dizziness, ataxia, blurred vision	Contraindications: Hypersensitivity to drug. Potential interactions: CNS depressants – ↑CNS depressant effects, Ketorolac – ↓anticonvulsant effect
Pregablin (Lyrica®)	Antiepileptic	Bind to voltage-gate calcium channels, and may modulate the release of excitatory neurotransmitters	50 mg TID, may titrate to 100 mg TID	Somnolence, dizziness, ataxia, blurred vision	Contraindications: Hypersensitivity to drug. Potential interactions: CNS depressants – ↑CNS depressant effects, Ketorolac – ↓anticonvulsant effect

(continued)

Table 10.2.   (continued)

Name	Drug class	Mode of action	Oral dosage	Main side effects	Important contraindications and potential interactions
Diazepam (Valium®)	Benzodiazepine	Binds to postsynaptic GABA neuron, enhancing the effector of GABA on neuronal excitability	2–8 mg PO qhs – BID	Vasodilation, depression, dizziness, headache, nausea	Contraindications: Hypersensitivity to drug, Narrow angle glaucoma Potential interactions: CNS depressants – ↑CNS depressant effect
Cyclobenzaprine (Flexeril®)	Skeletal muscle relaxant	Centrally acting skeletal muscle relaxant, reduces tonic somatic motor activity	5 mg TID, may titrate to 7.5–10 mg TID	Drowsiness, dizziness, xerostomia	Contraindications: Hypersensitivity to drug, MAO-I use within 14 days, hyperthyroidism, CHF, arrhythmias, recent MI Potential interactions: CNS depressants – ↑CNS depressant effect, MAO-I – serotonin syndrome, Anticholinergics – ↑ Anticholinergic effects

options, although numerous, must be tailored carefully to each individual patient. A single treatment regimen should be initiated, and then withheld, or added to, depending on effectiveness. Patient reassurance that they have an actual physical condition, and that it is not life-threatening, is vital when initiating therapy. A good doctor–patient relationship is paramount, as patients with this condition may be very frustrated from prior attempts at treatment. Initial medical management includes the following groups of drugs: antibiotics, alpha blockers, anti-inflammatories, 5-α reductase inhibitors, pain medications, and skeletal muscle relaxants (Table 10.2).

Antibiotics

Research into the use of antibiotics has not been promising for category III prostatitis, although antibiotics have worked well with category II prostatitis. Levofloxacin and ciprofloxacin showed no significant difference in efficacy when compared with placebo in men with CP/CPPS [9, 10]. Patients treated with 6 weeks of levofloxacin did have a greater decrease in symptoms as defined by the NIH-CPSI score. The general consensus in initial treatment for CP/CPPS is a 4–6 week trial of empiric antibiotics in antibiotic naïve individuals. It is important to avoid repeated courses of empiric antibiotics. Once the initial course is completed, further antibiotics are warranted if the urine culture is positive.

α Blockers (AB)

AB, such as alfuzosin and tamsulosin, are antagonists to the α adrenoceptors in the prostate and bladder neck and function to relax the smooth muscle, and have shown promise in the treatment of CP/CPPS. In a recent meta-analysis, AB showed a significant reduction in NIH-CPSI score and urinary symptom alleviation when used for more than 3 months [11]. AB did not show any benefit to pain in this analysis, however. In another study, when used for 6 weeks, tamsulosin was found to have a significant improvement in pain, urinary symptoms, and quality of life when compared with placebo [12]. Tamsulosin is usually well tolerated, and its efficacy increases with time. The combination of AB and antibiotics has not proven to be effective in recent clinical trials. A combination of ciprofloxacin and tamsulosin for 6 weeks did not substantially reduce symptoms in men with long-standing CP/CPPS who had at least moderate symptoms [10]. Levofloxacin was shown to be more effective for a 6-week short-term treatment of CP/CPPS than doxazosin alone or a combination of levofloxacin and doxazosin [13].

5α Reductase Inhibitors

Finasteride, a Type I 5-α reductase inhibitor, is an attractive medication to use in older men with CP/CPPS because it can be effective in treating concurrent symptoms of benign prostatic hyperplasia. In a prospective 1-year trial, finasteride was compared to saw palmetto in men with CP/CPPS. Finasteride yielded a significant decrease in NIH-CPSI score, where as patients treated with saw palmetto experienced no appreciable long-term improvement [14].

Other Medications

Other medications such as nonsteroidal anti-inflammatory drugs (NSAID), the bioflavinoid quercetin, and pentosan polysulfate have been shown to be effective by having anti-inflammatory properties. The COX-2 inhibitor refecoxib has also been shown to be effective in some men with CP/CPPS. The problem with these studies is that they were small and the results have not been subsequently reproduced.

Intuitively, medications that target neuropathic pain are thought to be of benefit in CP/CPPS, and indeed some are regularly used in clinical practice, as the main symptom is pain. Tricyclic antidepressant medications are used commonly for the treatment of neuropathic pain in chronic pain syndromes such as fibromyalgia. Tricyclics block the reuptake of norepinephrine and serotonin. It is believed that by blocking the reuptake of these neurotransmitters, their inhibitory effect on the central pain processing receptor is potentiated [15]. Nortriptyline is suggested to be the first-line tricyclic antidepressant, given its more favorable side effect profile, and starting doses should be 10 mg at bedtime, working up to a maximum of 75–100 mg at bedtime [16]. Gabapentin and pregablin are anticonvulsants that are also effective in treating neuropathic pain. Pregablin is currently under study in a randomized placebo-controlled trial for CP/CPPS. In severe cases of pain, refractory to non-addictive treatments, opioids may be warranted, but consultation with a pain specialist should be considered first.

Recognizing the symptoms of depression and anxiety in patients with CP/CPPS is crucial because psychiatric and somatic symptoms can cause a vicious cycle. A worsening psyche may cause worsening symptoms, and vice versa. Anti-anxiety and antidepressant medications should be used with assistance from a primary care physician or psychiatrist in the care of the patient. It is reasonable to discuss the possibility of psychiatric counseling with a patient if the physician feels that it may help in treatment.

Key Points

1. CP/CPPS is a complex condition that causes significant morbidity.
2. The etiology of CP/CPPS is unknown, and its diagnosis is one of exclusion; an appropriate work-up in patients with pelvic pain is required to rule out a potentially reversible cause.
3. Treatment strategies should be tailored to the patient, and multimodal therapy is usually required.
4. Avoid repeated courses of empiric antibiotics. Once the initial course is completed, further antibiotics are only warranted if the urine culture is positive.
5. Despite the name prostatitis, the predominant symptom is pelvic pain and therefore pain medications should be used to treat the symptoms.

References

1. Krieger JN, Nyberg L Jr, Nickel JC (1999) NIH consensus definition and classification of prostatitis. JAMA 282(3):236–237

2. True Ld, Berger RE, Rothman I et al (1999) Prostate histopathology and the chronic prostatitis/chronic pelvic pain syndrome: a prospective biopsy study. J Urol 162:2014–2018

3. Lee JC, Muller CH, Rothman I, et al (2003) Prostate biopsy culture findings of men with chronic pelvic pain syndrome do not differ from those of healthy controls [see comment]. J Urol 169(2):584–587 [discussion: 587–588]

4. Collins MM, Meigs JB, Barry MJ et al (2002) Prevalence and correlates of prostatitis in the health professionals follow-up study cohort. J Urol 167:1363–1366

5. Ishigooka M, Zermann DH, Doggweiler R et al (2000) Similarity of distributions of spinal c-Fos and plasma extravasation after acute chemical irritation of the bladder and the prostate. J Urol 164(5):1751–1756

6. Yang CC, Lee JC, Kromm BG, et al (2003) Pain sensitization in male chronic pelvic pain syndrome: why are symptoms so difficult to treat? J Urol 170(3):823 [discussion: 826–827]

7. Riley DE, Krieger JN (2002) X Chromosomal short tandem repeat polymorphisms near the phosphoglycerate kinase gene in men with chronic prostatitis. Biochim Biophys Acta 1586(1):99–107

8. Meares EM, Stamey TA (1968) Bacteriologic localization patterns in bacterial prostatitis and urethritis. Invest Urol 5(5):492–518

9. Nickel JC, Downey J, Clark J et al (2003) Levofloxacin for chronic prostatitis/chronic pelvic pain syndrome in men: a randomized placebo-controlled multicenter trial. Urology 62(4):614–617

10. Alexander RB, Propert KJ, Schaeffer AJ et al (2004) Ciprofloxacin or tamsulosin in men with chronic prostatitis/chronic pelvic pain syndrome: a randomized, double-blind trial. Ann Intern Med 141(8):581–589

11. Yang G, Wei Q, Li H et al (2006) The effect of α-adrenergic antagonist in chronic prostatis/chronic pelvic pain syndrome: a meta-analysis of randomized controlled trials. J Androl 27(6): 847–852

12. Nickel JC, Narayan P, McKay J, Doyle C (2004) Treatment of chronic prostatitis/chronic pelvic pain syndrome with tamsulosin: a randomized double blind trial. J Urol 171(4):1594–1597

13. Jeong CW, Lim DJ, Son H, Lee SE, Jeong H (2008) Treatment for chronic prostatitis/chronic pelvic pain syndrome: levofloxacin, doxazosin and their combination. Urol Int 80(2):157–161

14. Kaplan SA, Volpe MA, Te AE (2004) A prospective, 1-year trial using saw palmetto versus finasteride in the treatment of category III prostatitis/chronic pelvic pain syndrome. J Urol 171(1): 284–288

15. Godfrey RG (1996) A guide to the understanding and use of tricyclic antidepressants in the overall management of fibromyalgia and other chronic pain syndromes. Arch Intern Med 156:1047–1052

16. Dworkin RH, Backonja M, Rowbotham MC et al (2003) Advances in neuropathic pain: diagnosis, mechanisms, and treatment recommendations. Arch Neurol 60:1524–1534

Chapter 11
Urinary Tract Stones

William G. Robertson

Introduction

Since the era of predynastic Egypt until the present day, kidney stones have perplexed patients and physicians alike. Although since that time the methods for removing stones have advanced from the crudely barbaric to the highly sophisticated remedies of today, the problem of how successfully to prevent their recurrence continues to challenge both surgeons and physicians.

Urinary stone disease is a multi-factorial problem and there is no simple solution to the medical prevention of stone recurrence that will apply to all patients. To determine exactly which approach is necessary, the patient should first undergo a complete metabolic, nutritional, lifestyle, and epidemiological screen, such as that developed at University College Hospital and the Royal Free Hospital in London [1, 2]. From the resulting data, a complete profile of the risk factors leading to the cause of a particular patient's stone-formation can be identified and corrected.

W.G. Robertson (✉)
Department of Physiology, Centre for Nephrology, Royal Free and University College, London Medical School, London, NW3 2PF, UK

I.S. Shergill et al. (eds.), *Medical Therapy in Urology*,
DOI 10.1007/978-1-84882-704-2_11,
© Springer-Verlag London Limited 2010

Prevention of Stone Formation

If patients were not provided with appropriate preventative management, the risk of recurrence was traditionally high 40% within 3 years, rising to 74% at 10 years and to 98% at 25 years in the days when open surgery and transurethral basket or loop extraction were the main techniques for removing stones [3]. Since the introduction of extracorporeal shock-wave lithotripsy (ESWL) and percutaneous nephrolithotomy in the mid-1980s, the recurrence rate has become even higher, a fact that is not surprising as both techniques, particularly ESWL, often leave particles behind in the kidney that provide ideal nuclei for further stone-formation [4]. The recent introduction of flexible ureterenoscopy, however, may eventually lead to lower recurrence rates as this procedure is more likely to remove the entire stone, thereby reducing the risk of nucleation of new stones on fragments left behind after incomplete clearance of the urinary tract.

The main aim in the prevention of stone recurrence is to decrease the likelihood of crystals forming in the urinary tract by reducing the supersaturation of urine with respect to the particular constituent/constituents that occurs/occur in the patients' stones. In some patients, treatment may be helped by increasing the ability of urine to inhibit the crystallization of the calcium salts that constitute the majority of urinary stones.

A summary of the available dietary and medical treatments for the various types of urinary calculi is shown in Table 11.1. Although most of these are effective in reducing the risk of stone recurrence, the main problem in the long-term management of stone patients is compliance [5]. Generally, stone-formers feel well for most of the time, except when they experience an attack of renal colic. It is often difficult, therefore, to maintain their cooperation and motivation to adhere to their preventative treatment over a long period after their stone episode. If they do not have a recurrence of their problem within a few months of their episode, most stone-formers will regress to their original abnormal pattern of urine biochemistry within 3–6 months and will eventually produce more stones [5]. Once they have had several episodes

TABLE 11.1.   Summary of medical methods for prevention
of urinary stone disease.

Stone type	Treatment
2,8-Dihydroxyadenine	Very high fluid intake (>3 l/day) + allopurinol (300 mg/day)
Silica	Discontinue magnesium trisilicate antacids
Xanthine	Hereditary form: high fluid intake + oral alkali (urine pH >7.4) Iatrogenic form: withdraw allopurinol
Cystine stones	Very high fluid intake (>3 l/day) + oral alkali (urine pH >7.5) or D-penicillamine (2–4 g/day) or α-mercaptopropionylglycine (0.8–1.2 g/day)
Uric acid stones	High fluid intake (>2.5 l/day) + oral alkali (urine pH >6.2) or allopurinol (300 mg/day) or reduce purine intake
Ammonium urate stones	Laxative abuse: advise patient to stop taking laxatives Urinary tract infection: treat with antibiotics
Infected stones	High fluid intake + antibiotics + oral acid (pH <6.2)
Calcium stones	
Idiopathic	High fluid intake + dietary advice or thiazide diuretics (bendrofluazide 10 mg/day) or magnesium supplements (500 mg/day) or potassium citrate (20 mequiv tds)
Hyperparathyroid	Parathyroidectomy or, if contraindicated, high fluids + oral acid
Hereditary hyperoxaluric	High fluid intake (>3 l/day) + pyridoxine (300 mg/day)
Enteric hyperoxaluric	High fluid intake + low oxalate/high calcium diet or potassium citrate
Renal tubular acidotic	High fluid intake + thiazides or potassium citrate
Medullary sponge kidney	Treat as for idiopathic
Corticosteroid-induced	Discontinue corticosteroids: treat as for idiopathic
Sarcoidosis	High fluid intake
Milk-alkali syndrome	Discontinue alkali and moderate calcium intake + high fluid intake
Vitamin D intoxication	Discontinue high vitamin D intake + high fluid intake

(continued)

TABLE 11.1.   (continued)

Stone type	Treatment
Betel-nut chewing	Discontinue practice
Immobilization	High fluid intake; remobilize as far as possible; treat any urinary tract infection with antibiotics
Antacid abuse	Discontinue calcium-containing antacids; change to proton pump inhibitors
Tropical holidays	Protect skin from UV radiation + increase fluid intake (not more alcohol) while on holiday
Dietary excesses	Reduce intake of animal protein and/or sodium and/or refined sugars and/or oxalate and/or calcium as necessary
Dietary deficiencies	Increase intake of fluid and/or fresh fruit and vegetables and/or brown bread, brown pasta, brown rice, and breakfast cereals as necessary
Iatrogenic stones	Discontinue drug concerned as far as possible and replace with alternative therapy + high fluid intake

of renal colic, it is usually easier to motivate them on a more continuous basis.

It is important to review the patient regularly as an outpatient and to repeat the 24-h Urine screen tests [6], preferably annually but at least biennially, to ensure that they are adhering to the prophylaxis prescribed and to check that their biochemical risk of stones remains low [7].

Medical Therapies in Urinary Tract Stones

The list of common medical treatments in urinary tract stone disease is listed in Table 11.2, and below, each type of stone is discussed with regard to the medical therapies available.

Calcium Stones

Calcium stone-formation is by far the most common form of the disorder accounting for around 80% of all stone-formers.

TABLE 11.2.   Medical therapies in urinary tract stone disease.

Name	Mode of action	Oral dosage	Main side effects	Important contraindications and potential interactions
Bendrofluazide	Increases the tubular reabsorption of calcium, which, through a feedback mechanism, leads to a reduction in the intestinal absorption and urinary excretion of calcium	10 mg/day		The limitation of this form of treatment is the amount of magnesium that can be given without causing intestinal discomfort and diarrhoea
Magnesium supplements	Magnesium forms a soluble complex with oxalate in the gut and reduces oxalate absorption in the colon. It also reduces the concentration of "free" ionized oxalate available for precipitation with calcium in urine	500 mg/day	Intestinal discomfort and diarrhoea	
Potassium citrate [18]	Increases the urinary excretion of citrate (which is an inhibitor of the crystallization of calcium salts in urine). It also decreases the urinary excretion of calcium by increasing its tubular reabsorption through its alkalinizing effect on urine	20 mequiv tds		Alkalinization increases the supersaturation of calcium phosphate and some patients can be converted from forming CaOx stones to CaP stones

(continued)

TABLE 11.2.   (continued)

Name	Mode of action	Oral dosage	Main side effects	Important contraindications and potential interactions
Pyridoxine	This reduces the metabolic production of oxalate in about a third of patients with primary hyperoxaluria (type 1) and in a few patients with mild hyperoxaluria	300 mg/day		Neurological problems with high dosage
Allopurinol	Inhibits Xanthine oxidase inhibitor its concentration in urine	400 mg/d		Caution in patients who have a very high production of uric acid (Lesch–Nyhan syndrome or neoplastic disease) since allopurinol administration may result in xanthinuria and xanthine stones
D-Penicillamine	Chelating agent that combines with cystine to form a soluble disulfide complex. The D-penicillamine–cysteine complex is much more soluble in urine than cystine and is excreted harmlessly in urine	2–4 g/day	Rash, arthralgia, nephritic syndrome and gastrointestinal disturbance	Previous hypersensitivity; penicillamine-related agranulocytosis or aplastic anemia

Thiola, N-Acetyl-D-Penicillamine [8]	Chelating agent that combines with cystine to form a soluble disulfide complex		Previous hypersensitivity; agranulocytosis or aplastic anemia
α-Mercaptopropionylglycine [9]	Chelating agent that combines with cystine to form a soluble disulfide complex	250 mg/d	Lower side effects thank D-Penicillamine
Tamsulosin (Flomax®)	Inhibits α1a-receptors in the prostate and bladder neck, causing smooth muscle relaxation and improvement of urine flow (selective α-blockade)	0.4 mg Q HS (can titrate to 0.8 mg Q HS)	Orthostatic hypotension, headache, dizziness, abnormal ejaculation; Contraindications: hypersensitivity to drug; Potential Interactions: β-blocker → ↑orthostatic effects

About 12% of all calcium stone-formers have an underlying metabolic cause of their stones; the remainder are so-called idiopathic. The stones themselves can occur in a number of forms – mixed calcium oxalate/uric acid stones, pure calcium oxalate stones, mixed calcium oxalate/calcium phosphate stones, and pure calcium phosphate stones. The risk of forming each type of stone may be estimated from an analysis of the patient's 24-h urine [5].

Calcium oxalate (CaOx) is the most insoluble of all the stone-forming salts and acids and it is the constituent of stones of which normal subjects are most at risk of precipitating in their urine. However, stone-formers have higher urinary supersaturation levels with respect to calcium salts than normal subjects and form crystals more frequently and of greater size than do normal subjects. Once a CaOx-containing stone has formed, it is almost impossible to dissolve it in situ.

The main urinary risk factors for the formation of calcium-containing stones are, in decreasing order of importance: a low urine volume, mild hyperoxaluria, an increase in urinary pH, hypercalciuria, hypocitraturia, hypomagnesiuria, and hyperuricosuria [5]. In most patients, there is often no single obvious urinary abnormality that is the cause of the stone: usually the stones are due to a combination of a number of small changes in urine composition, which together cause the patient to be at an increased overall biochemical risk of forming stones. The importance of mild hyperoxaluria should not be overlooked. It is often not measured at all or is unreliable owing to poor oxalate measurement in urine.

There are various means of preventing the recurrence of calcium-containing stones, and these are described below:

1. High fluid intake, enough to produce at least 2.5 l/day of urine under all circumstances, works by diluting the urinary concentrations of calcium, oxalate, and phosphate [8].
2. Thiazide diuretics (Bendrofluazide 10 mg/day) in order to increase the tubular reabsorption of calcium, which, through a feedback mechanism, leads to a reduction in the intestinal absorption and urinary excretion of calcium [9].

3. Magnesium supplements (500 mg additional mg/day). Magnesium forms a soluble complex with oxalate in the gut and reduces oxalate absorption in the colon. It also reduces the concentration of "free" ionized oxalate available for pre-cipitation with calcium in urine. The limitation of this form of treatment is the amount of magnesium that can be given without causing intestinal discomfort and diarrhoea [10].

4. Potassium citrate (20 mequiv tds). This is a popular form of treatment in the USA and is designed to increase the urinary excretion of citrate [11]. Citrate is an inhibitor of the crystallization of calcium salts in urine. It also decreases the urinary excretion of calcium by increasing its tubular reabsorption through its alkalinizing effect on urine. The main disadvantage of this form of treatment is that the alkalinization increases the supersaturation of urine with respect to calcium phosphate and some patients can be converted from forming CaOx stones to CaP stones. Also, potassium citrate does not always increase the urinary excretion of citrate, particularly in patients with the severe hypocitraturia found in distal renal tubular acidosis.

5. Pyridoxine (300 mg/day). This reduces the metabolic pro-duction of oxalate in about a third of patients with primary hyperoxaluria (type 1) and in a few patients with mild hyperoxaluria. However, there may be some neurological problems with this high dosage [12].

6. Correction of dietary extremes [13]. Dietary extremes explain much of the changing pattern of stone incidence over the past 100 years. As the composition of the national diet has become "richer" owing to an increased consump-tion of protein (particularly animal protein), fat, refined sugars, and salt (the so-called "bad Western diet"), the inci-dence of stones has increased. This often follows periods of economic expansion. During periods of recession, on the other hand, the incidence of stones has been noted to decrease in parallel with a return to a more healthy form of diet containing more fresh fruit and vegetables, more fiber and fewer energy-rich foods. In some patients, a high dietary intake of calcium or oxalate may also have to be corrected.

Uric Acid Stones

The majority of these stones are attributable to some metabolic disorder, which leads to a high excretion of uric acid in urine and/or a persistently acid urine, with a $pH < 5.5$ [14]. As with all types of urolithiasis, a low urine volume increases the risk of crystalluria and stone-formation. All three factors are important in the genesis of uric acid stones. Treatment is designed to lower the supersaturation of urine with respect to uric acid by correcting the urinary risk factors for uric acid stones (hyperuricosuria, a persistently acid urine, or a highly concentrated urine).

1. Alkali combined with a high fluid intake is the easiest form of treatment to keep urinary pH above 6.2 (but not >6.5 to avoid the risk of forming calcium phosphate stones) with oral sodium bicarbonate or potassium citrate and maintaining the urine volume above 2.5 l/day with a high fluid intake.
2. Allopurinol, which inhibits the metabolic production of uric acid from xanthine, is useful in many cases of hyperurico-suria due to metabolic over-production [15]. It has few side effects, but care has to be taken with patients who have a very high production of uric acid (such as in Lesch–Nyhan syndrome or neoplastic disease) since allopurinol admin-istration may result in xanthinuria and xanthine stones. It may also be useful in patients who cannot tolerate alkali.
3. Dietary hyperuricosuria due to excessive purine ingestion can be treated simply by reducing the intake of high purine foods (mainly meat, fish and poultry and pulses, such as peas and beans).

Infection Stones

These stones, which generally consist of calcium phosphate (CaP) and/or magnesium ammonium phosphate (MAP), are often large (staghorn calculi) and are secondary to a urinary tract infection with a urea-splitting organism. These organisms contain the enzyme, urease, which can break down urea to ammonia, bicarbonate, and hydroxyl ions [16]. This produces urine that is very alkaline and contains an unphysiologically high concentration of ammonium ions for such alkaline urine. These conditions are ideal for the precipitation of CaP and MAP. Urine of normal subjects is generally well undersaturated with respect to MAP and so they are at no risk of MAP crystalluria.

Infection stones are more common in women than in men. It should be noted that a proportion of stone-formers develop a urinary tract infection secondary to their original sterile stone of a totally different composition. So that sometimes the MAP and CaP can form on top of other calculi. In these cases, there is usually an underlying set of problems that led to the original sterile stone, and these have to be investigated.

Treatment of infection stones requires antibiotic therapy to control the underlying infection [17]. However, it is often extremely difficult to eradicate the infection completely, particularly if the stones and/or their fragments, which may continue to harbor live micro-organisms, are not completely removed.

Cystine Stones

Normal subjects excrete very low concentrations of cystine in their urine, well below the precipitation point for this amino acid. Patients with cystinuria, an autosomal recessive disorder caused by a defect in the renal tubular transport mechanism for reabsorbing cystine, ornithine, lysine and arginine, excrete much higher concentrations of the amino acid [6]. Heterozygotes, in general, do not excrete quite enough cystine to cause cystine crystalluria and rarely form cystine-containing stones. Homozygotes, however, excrete much more cystine than the heterozygotes and regularly pass crystals of cystine in their urine. They form cystine stones usually from childhood but it is not unknown for the onset of stones to be delayed until adulthood.

There is no known cure for the underlying renal tubular defect, although conceivably advancements in genetic engineering may eventually allow the abnormal gene(s) to be corrected. Currently, treatment has to be directed at reducing the urinary concentration of the undissociated, acidic form of cystine below the precipitation point for the acid in urine. At urine pH vales below 7.4, this usually requires reducing the concentration of undissociated cystine to <0.6 mmol/l. Above pH 7.5, the target may be raised to <0.8 mmol/l. The methods used to achieve these targets are:

1. High fluid intake, but this must be enough to produce a 24-h urine volume >3 l/day. This relies solely on diluting the undissociated cystine concentration in urine to a point where cystine cannot precipitate spontaneously.
2. Alkali, enough to keep urinary pH above 7.5. This relies on causing the dissociation of the acidic form of cystine to the more soluble cystinate ion.
3. D-Penicillamine (2–4 g/day). This is expensive and can cause a number of severe side-effects. It is a chelating agent that combines with cystine to form a soluble disulfide complex. The D-penicillamine– cysteine complex is much more soluble in urine than cystine and is excreted harmlessly in urine [7].
4. Thiola, N-Acetyl-D-Penicillamine [18], and α-Mercaptopropionylglycine [19] are all less toxic than D-penicillamine, but act in the same way to form soluble complexes with the cysteine subunits of cystine, which are then excreted safely in urine.

Xanthine Stones

There are three situations that lead to an increased excretion of xanthine in the urine and about 30% of patients with this urinary abnormality form stones. These stones are very rare in the West and are usually secondary to Allopurinol administration in patients with very high uric acid production rates, such as in Lesch–Nyhan Syndrome or in neoplastic disease. Allopurinol is a xanthine oxidase inhibitor and its administration may lead to a build-up of xanthine, which is excreted in the urine. The second cause is molybdenum deficiency and the third cause is a rare hereditary disorder of purine metabolism, probably autosomal recessive in nature, which is characterized by a deficiency of xanthine oxidase.

1. Treatment of xanthine stone-formation involves aggressive alkali therapy in order to solubilize the xanthine, but this is even more difficult than in the case of cystinuria. A high fluid intake will help but requires a urine volume of more than 3–5 l/day.
2. Cases of hereditary xanthinuria can be treated with Allopurinol in order to block the residual oxidation of hypoxanthine to xanthine. The resulting increase in hypoxanthine is unimportant as it is relatively soluble in urine.
3. The iatrogenic form of the disorder can be treated by discontinuing the administration of Allopurinol.

2,8-Dihydroxyadenine (2,8-DHA) Stones

This occurs in patients with a rare inborn error of purine metabolism in which there is a deficiency of the adenine salvage enzyme adenine phosphoribosyltransferase. This leads to a high excretion of 2,8-DHA in urine where it is insoluble. Allopurinol is an effective treatment for this disorder since it prevents the production of 2,8-DHA and so reduces its concentration in urine.

Silica Stones

Although relatively common in grazing animals, these stones are rare in man. They usually occur secondarily to the ingestion of magnesium trisilicate-containing antacids, which, in some patients, lead to a high excretion of silica in urine. These stones can be prevented by changing to another form of antacid treatment.

Ammonium Urate Stones

Laxative abuse may cause ammonium urate stones to form by decreasing urine volume and urinary citrate and increasing ammonium ion excretion [20]. Treatment involves persuading the patient to stop taking laxatives. Occasionally, ammonium urate is found in stones from patients with urinary tract infections. Treatment involves elimination of the urinary tract infection with antibiotics.

Iatrogenic Stones

Some stones, like those consisting of silica mentioned above, can form following the administration of a drug, which itself is either insoluble in urine or one of its metabolites is insoluble in urine. Examples include: sulfonamide antibiotics, triamterene, and indinavir (used in the treatment of HIV Aids). Ascorbic acid (vitamin C), piridoxilate, and methoxyflurane anesthetic all increase the urinary excretion of oxalate and so increase the risk of calcium oxalate stone-formation. Glycine irrigation during transurethral prostatectomy may lead to calcium oxalate crystalluria, which is a major risk factor for stone-formation. Treatment involves a high fluid intake and/or changing to an alternative form of medication for the disorder concerned.

Key Points

1. Urinary stone disease is a multi-factorial problem and there is no simple solution to the medical prevention of stone recurrence that will apply to all patients.
2. For most patients, a high fluid intake, sufficient consistently to produce 2.5 l of urine per day (with the exception of cystine stone-formers who require to produce >3 l/day), will reduce their risk of forming further stones.
3. For some, however, additional measures are required to correct their metabolic and/or dietary abnormalities.
4. To determine exactly which approach is necessary, the patient should first undergo a complete metabolic, nutritional, lifestyle, and epidemiological screen.
5. From the resulting data, a complete profile of the risk factors leading to the cause of a particular patient's stone-formation can be identified and corrected.

References

1. Robertson WG (2000) Predicting the outcome of the medical management of stone-formers by risk factor analysis. In: Rodgers AL, Hibbert BE, Hess B, Khan SR, Preminger GM (eds) Urolithiasis 2000. University of Cape Town Press, Cape Town, pp 533–534

2. Robertson WG (2003) A risk factor model of stone-formation. Front Biosci 8:1330–1338

3. Williams RE (1963) Long-term survey of 538 patients with upper urinary tract stone. B J Urol 35:416–437

4. Robertson WG (1998) The medical management of urinary stone disease. Europ Urol Update Series 7:139–144

5. Norman RW, Bath SS, Robertson WG, Peacock M (1984) When should patients with symptomatic stone disease be evaluated metabolically? J Urol 132:1137–1139

6. Dent CE, Senior B, Walshe JM (1954) The pathogenesis of cystinuria. II. Polarographic studies of the metabolism of sulphur-containing amino acids. J Clin Invest 33:1216–1226

7. Crawhall JC, Scowen EF, Watts RWE (1963) Effect of penicillamine on cystinuria. B Med J 1:588–590

8. Pak CYC, Sakhaee K, Crowther C, Brinkley L (1980) Evidence justifying a high fluid intake in treatment of nephrolithiasis. Ann Intern Med 93:36–39

9. Yendt ER, Cohanim M (1978) Prevention of renal stones with thiazides. Kidney Int 13:397–409

10. Lindberg J, Harvey J, Pak CYC (1990) Effect of magnesium citrate and magnesium oxide on the crystallisation of calcium salts in urine; changes produced by food – magnesium interaction. J Urol 143:248–251

11. Fine JK, Pak CYC, Preminger GM (1995) Effect of medical management and residual fragments on recurrent stone formation following shock wave lithotripsy. J Urol 153:27–33

12. Smith LH, Williams HE (1967) Treatment of primary hyperoxaluria. Mod Treat 4:522–530

13. Robertson WG (1987) Diet and calcium stones. Miner Electrolyte Metab 13:228–234

14. Metcalfe-Gibson A, MacCallum FM, Morrison RBI, Wrong O (1965) Urinary excretion of hydrogen ion in patients with uric acid calculi. Clin Sci 28:325–345

15. Godfrey RG, Rankin TJ (1969) Uric acid renal lithiasis: management by allopurinol. J Urol 101:643–647

16. Lerner SP, Gleeson MJ, Griffith DP (1989) Infection stones. J Urol 141:753–758

17. Chinn RH, Maskell R, Mead JE, Polak A (1976) Renal stone and urinary infection: a study of antibiotic treatment. B Med J 2:1411–1413

18. Stokes GS, Potts JT, Lotz M, Bartter FC (1968) New agent in the treatment of cystinuria: N-acetyl-D-penicillamine. B Med J 1:284–288

19. Pak CYC, Sakhaee FC, Zerwekh JE K, Adams BV (1986) Management of cystine nephrolithiasis with α-mercaptopropionylglycine. J Urol 136:1003–1008

20. Dick WH, Lingeman JE, Preminger GM, Smith LH, Wilson DM, Shirrell WL (1990) Laxative abuse as a cause of ammonium urate renal calculi. J Urol 143:244–247

Chapter 12
Erectile Dysfunction

Chi-Ying Li and David Ralph

Introduction

Erectile dysfunction (ED) is defined as the consistent inability to achieve or maintain an erection. This may affect around 50% of men between the ages of 40 and 70, while persistent ED affects about 5% of men in their 40s, and 15–25% of men by the age of 65 [1]. As life expectancy increases, the incidence of ED is expected to rise.

Physiology of Erection

To understand the mechanisms underlying the medical management of ED, one must appreciate the physiological process of erection, as the medical therapies are designed to target certain parts of the cellular mechanisms, to achieve erection.

The process of erection is initiated through two main categories of stimuli, namely psychogenic and reflexogenic. Psychogenic erections are initiated in the supraspinal centers in the brain, in response to various visual, olfactory, and auditory stimuli, while reflexogenic erections are elicited by stimulation of receptors in the glans penis via the sensory afferent of the penis, known as the dorsal nerve [2]. Both mechanisms interact and are

C.-Y. Li (✉)
Department of Urology, Princess Alexandra Hospital, NHS Trust, Essex, UK

I.S. Shergill et al. (eds.), *Medical Therapy in Urology*,
DOI 10.1007/978-1-84882-704-2_12,
© Springer-Verlag London Limited 2010

coordinated through the sympathetic and parasympathetic outflow at the level of the spinal cord. During resting conditions, the sympathetic tone maintains the penis in a flaccid state. With the initiation of the process of erection, via the stimuli mentioned above, the parasympathetic system is activated, which results in the release of neurotransmitters, including acetylcholine and nitric oxide (NO). After release, NO activates soluble guanylate cyclase (GC), an enzyme, which in turn converts guanosine triphosphate (GTP) to cyclic guanosine monophosphate (cGMP). There are other neurotransmitters, the most important of these being prostaglandin E1 (PGE1), which via a different second messenger pathway, activates adenylyl cyclase, an enzyme which converts adenosine triphosphate (ATP) to cyclic adenosine monophosphate (cAMP). This, like cGMP, acts as a second messenger, in turn leading to changes in intracellular calcium, and thus there is smooth muscle relaxation in both the vascular endothelium in the penis as well as the corporal smooth muscle itself. The resultant effect is a significant increase in blood flow to the penis and erection ensues. The intracellular levels of cGMP and cAMP are finely tuned by a group of enzymes, known as the phosphodiesterases (PDE). In human corpus cavernosum, PDE2, 4, and 5 are present. Three of the current oral pharmacotherapy agents act by inhibiting this enzyme, known as the PDE5 inhibitors; these act by inhibiting PDE5 enzyme, which itself breaks down cGMP. Thus, inhibiting the action of PDE5 decreases the degradation of cGMP and increases the intracellular concentration of cGMP, enhancing the process of erection. Other medical therapies, namely PGE1 analogs, act via the effects of the prostaglandin pathway.

The mechanism of the process of erection is summarized in Fig. 12.1.

Etiology

Various etiological factors have been demonstrated to be associated with ED. More commonly, a combination of these causes contributes to the etiology of ED and overall 75–80% of ED is caused by vascular or neural disorders or a combination of both (Table 12.1).

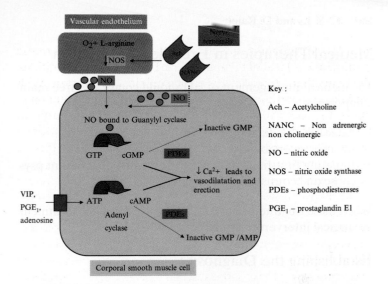

FIGURE 12.1. Diagram showing the intracellular physiological processes leading to erection

TABLE 12.1. Etiology of erectile dysfunction (ED).

Causes	Risk factors/conditions
Vasculogenic	Endothelial dysfunction [21] – hypertension, smoking, hypercholesterolemia, and diabetes Nitric oxide (NO) deficiency – atherosclerosis, diabetes, and aging Veno-occlusive dysfunction – characterized by venous insufficiency, despite adequate arterial inflow
Neurogenic	Parkinson's, Alzheimer's disease, cerebral vascular accident, multiple sclerosis, head injury, tumor, temporal lobe epilepsy, and peripheral neuropathy, e.g., diabetic autonomic neuropathy and Vitamin B deficiency in chronic alcoholism
Endocrine	Metabolic syndrome/hypogonadism, hyperprolactinemia, hyper- or hypothyroidism
Anatomical	Post prostatectomy (radical/TURP) Abdominal or pelvic surgery – abdomino-perineal resection, aorto-iliac bypass and pelvic radiotherapy Spinal cord injury/trauma
Drugs	Thiazide diuretics – spironolactone Centrally acting – alpha-methyldopa, reserpine, chlorpromazine, haloperidol, cimetidine, and verapamil Cocaine
Psychogenic	Stress, anxiety, and depression

Medical Therapies in Erectile Dysfunction

The medical management of ED should comprise three main components:

1. Establish the diagnosis.
2. Identify reversible risk factors, which can be treated.
3. Initiating first-line medical therapy, with concomitant psychosexual counseling if indicated.

When these treatments have failed, then second-line treatment or surgical intervention may be considered.

Establishing the Diagnosis

When assessing patients presenting with ED, the most important factor in successful management is a careful medical and detailed sexual history. This enables an accurate diagnosis of ED and establishes a possible underlying cause. It is also important to identify patients' concerns and expectations; this allows the treatment plan to be tailored to the specific needs of each patient. Where possible, the patients' partner should also be involved; taking into consideration both the patients' and the partners' preferences and expectations.

Identify Reversible Risk Factors, Which Can Be Treated

Recent studies [3–5] have demonstrated that various cardiovascular risk factors have been shown to be associated with ED.

The most important finding is that ED may constitute part of a more generalized disease of endothelial dysfunction and presents before other cardiovascular diseases with a lead time in onset of symptoms. This lead time in clinical presentation may be utilized in detecting otherwise asymptomatic and more sinister underlying cardiovascular conditions [6, 7].

Consequently, current recommendations in the management of ED concentrate on the screening and prevention of other cardiovascular diseases as well as treating the ED itself.

The current recommendations from the British Society of Sexual Medicine state that all patients should be screened for cardiovascular risk factors [8].

These include a thorough physical examination including assessment of blood pressure, heart rate, weight, and waist circumference. All patients should have their serum fasting glucose, lipids, and morning testosterone measured, to detect otherwise undiagnosed diabetes, hyperlipidemia, and hypogonadism, as ED associated with hypogonadism is potentially reversible with supplementary testosterone [9]. Patients with cardiovascular risk factors are then stratified into three groups (Table 12.2): low, intermediate, and high risks. Those in the intermediate and high-risk groups should be referred for specialist investigations.

Medical Therapies

Initiation with a single first-line agent should be considered in those patients with a normal level of testosterone; once they have had their cardiovascular risk factors stratified and are deemed safe to be started on treatment.

Current medical treatment options for ED are described in Table 12.3 and can be divided into the following categories:

1. Oral pharmacological agents
   (a) Sildenafil [Viagra®]
   (b) Tadalafil [Cialis®]
   (c) Vardenafil [Levitra®]
2. Injection therapy
   (a) Intracavernosal Alprostadil [Caverject®, Viridal®]
   (b) Intraurethral Alprostadil [MUSE®]

Oral Pharmacological Agents

An ideal treatment option for ED should be simple to use, convenient for the patient, not invasive, have minimal side effects and consistent efficacy. With the above criteria in mind, it is not hard to imagine that oral pharmacological agents are the most widely accepted form of treatment for ED and are therefore commonly used as the first-line agent.

TABLE 12.2.   Risk stratification, according to cardiovascular risk factors, of patients with ED.

Risk status	Variables	Management strategy
Low	Controlled hypertension <3 risk factors for coronary artery disease (excluding age and sex) Mild valvular disease Minimal/mild stable angina and following successful revascularization	Primary care
Medium	>3 risk factors for coronary artery disease (excluding age and sex) Moderate stable angina Recent myocardial infarction (MI) (<6 weeks) Congestive heart failure Murmur of unknown cause and noncardiac cause of atherosclerotic disease including peripheral vascular diseases History of CVA or TIA	Refer for specialist investigations including exercise treadmill test or echocardiogram Treatment for ED may be initiated depending on the results of the investigations
High	Recent MI or cerebral vascular event (<2 weeks) Uncontrolled hypertension (systolic BP>180) Unstable angina Moderate to severe valve disease High-risk arrhythmias Obstructive hypertrophic cardiomyopathies	Patients in this group should not have treatment for ED until specialist investigation has been completed

TABLE 12.3. Medical therapy of ED.

Drug	Mode of action	Dose	Common side effects	Interactions and contraindications
Sildenafil [Viagra®]	PDE5 inhibitor	25 mg; 50 mg; 100 mg	Dyspepsia, vomiting, headache, flushing, dizziness, visual disturbances, raised intraocular pressure, nasal congestion, back pain, myalgia, hypertension/ hypotension, syncope, photosensitivity	Patients receiving nitrates or patients in whom vasodilatation or sexual activity are inadvisable Hypotension, recent MI, unstable angina and stroke (<6 weeks) Hereditary degenerative retinal disorders
Tadalafil [Cialis®]	PDE5 inhibitor	10 mg; 20 mg	As above for sildenafil Dyspepsia, vomiting, headache, flushing, dizziness, visual disturbances, raised intraocular pressure, nasal congestion, back pain, myalgia, hypertension/ hypotension, syncope, photosensitivity	Caution in anatomical deformation of the penis, including penile curvature/Peyronie's disease and in those with a predisposition to prolonged erection Acute postural hypotension has been reported in sildenafil treatment combined with doxazosin. Sildenafil >25 mg should not be taken within 4 h of alpha-blockers The recommendation for using alpha-blockers with tadalafil and vardenafil is to exercise caution Itraconazole, ketaconazole

(continued)

TABLE 12.3.   (continued)

Drug	Mode of action	Dose	Common side effects	Interactions and contraindications
Vardenafil [Levitra®]	PDE5 inhibitor	5 mg; 10 mg; 20 mg	As above for sildenafil	Protease inhibitors e.g., Indinavir and Ritonavir
Alprostadil [Caverject®]	Prostaglandin E1 analog	5 mcg; 10 mcg; 20 mcg	Hypotension, hypertension, injection sites – infection, bleeding, penile hematoma, and cavernosal fibrosis	Sickle cell anemia, multiple myeloma, leukemia, or patients with penile implant
Alprostadil [Viridal®]	Prostaglandin E1 analog	10 mcg; 20 mcg; 40 mcg	Priapism	
Intraurethral [MUSE®]	Prostaglandin E1 analog	250 mcg (titrate to response <1 mg)	Urethral burning/bleeding Priapism	Urethral stricture, severe penile curvature Balanitis, urethritis

The first-line agents are the PDE5 inhibitors, namely sildenafil [Viagra®], tadalafil [Cialis®], and vardenafil [Levitra®]. These agents act by inhibiting PDE5 enzymes, thus increasing the intracellular concentration of cGMP and enhancing the process of erection, as discussed above.

There are currently no double blind randomized control trials directly comparing the efficacy of these agents with each other, although all have been proven to be superior to placebo [10–12], including specific "difficult to treat" subgroups, in particular those with diabetes and post radical prostatectomy surgery. They are generally well tolerated. Despite the relative controversy over the efficacies of these agents, the characteristics of each agent are widely accepted. The significant differences between these drugs are discussed below and tabulated in Table 12.4.

Sildenafil [Viagra®] and vardenafil [Levitra®] have a relatively short half life of approximately 4 h, whereas tadalafil [Cialis®] has a slightly longer half life of 17.5 h. Therefore, in patients suffering from side effects, a slightly shorter acting agent may be considered. Tadalafil [Cialis®] and vardenafil [Levitra®] should be taken between approximately 30 min and 2 h before sexual intercourse is attempted, while sildenafil [Viagra®] should be taken 60 min before. These properties can be used to suit patients' individual sexual practices. Interaction with food is greatest with sildenafil [Viagra®] and least with tadalafil [Cialis®]. Vardenafil [Levitra®] has pharmacologically the lowest concentration required to achieve 50% smooth muscle relaxation, thus theoretically the lowest drug concentration required to achieve smooth muscle relaxation and erection.

These characteristics may be used in deciding which agent should be initiated in each patient, and all men should be informed of these drug characteristics, the dosing regime, and be given adequate opportunity to trial different options, before deciding which option best suits their needs, depending on the requisites and constraints of each occasion.

Should patients fail to respond to initial monotherapy with PDE5 treatment, several salvage approaches should be considered. These include ensuring adequate patient education on

TABLE 12.4.   The pharmacokinetics of oral phosphodiesterase type 5 (PDE5) inhibitors.

	Sildenafil [Viagra®]	Tadalafil [Cialis®]	Vardenafil [Levitra®]
Maximum plasma concentration Minutes	30–120 (median 60)	30–360 (median 120)	30–120 (median 60)
Half life Hours	4	17.5	4–5
Duration of action Hours	Up to 4–12	Up to 36	Up to 4–12
Food restriction	May take longer to work with meals	Can be taken with or without food	Can be taken with or without fatty food

the dosing regime and characteristics of PDE5 inhibitors, regular evaluation, and correction of risk factors, trial of another PDE5 inhibitor; occasionally, patients may respond to another PDE5 inhibitor.

It is important to appreciate that efficacy for one agent does not necessarily imply patient preference and the greatest factor in achieving success in management of ED is patient education, as these considerations have been demonstrated to improve PDE5 inhibitor treatment response rates [13–15].

If a patient fails the initial treatment, a second-line agent should be considered. It is currently recommended that PDE5 nonresponders are defined as patients who have failed to respond to >8 doses, at the highest tolerated dosage, of preferably two different PDE5 inhibitors, taken sequentially.

Of note, other oral sublingual pharmacotherapy includes Apomorphine [Uprima®], which is a centrally acting, non-opioid dopaminergic receptor agonist. This was discontinued in the UK in 2006. Previous studies reported an efficacy rate of 26–32%, comparing less favorably to sildenafil. Apomorphine differs from PDE5 inhibitors in that it is tolerated in patients receiving nitrates. However, caution should be exercised in patients suffering from ischemic heart disease where hypotension is not advised.

ED treatment may be prescribed in the NHS with "SLS" (selected list scheme, this is a list of items agreed by the Department of Health to be funded by the NHS) endorsed on the prescription, but these are limited to patients with certain medical conditions or patients where ED causes a significant disruption to normal activities, marked effect on mood, behavior, social and environmental awareness, or a marked effect on interpersonal relationship [16].

Injection Therapy – Intracavernosal or Intraurethral Options

These agents may be used as first-line treatment for patients where PDE5 inhibitors are contraindicated, or more commonly as a second-line regime, due to their invasive nature, for those who have failed PDE5 treatments. Alprostadil, a

PGE1 analog [Caverject®, Viridal®], is given as an intracavernosal injection or via intraurethral [MUSE®] placement to induce an erection. PGE1 acts via activation of adenylyl cyclase, which converts ATP to cAMP as discussed above.

Patients self-inject Caverject® or Viridal® intracavernosally after an initial demonstration by a heathcare professional. In patients where self-injection is problematic, partners may be involved and taught to give the injections. The initial dose is 2.5 mcg, followed by increments of 5–10 mcg, until a satisfactory response for an erection lasting for no more than 1 h.

Intracavernosal injections have a high efficacy rate with reported erection enabling sexual activity in up to 80% of injections with an 80–90% sexual satisfaction rate [17].

There are reported complications associated with injection sites, including bleeding, penile hematoma, infection, and cavernosal fibrosis. Patients must be warned of the risk of priapism and should seek medical help if prolonged unwanted erection develops or for erection lasting for more than 4 h.

Intraurethral alprostadil [MUSE®] involves patients placing the prostaglandin pellet urethrally via the use of an applicator and the penis is then massaged to encourage delivery of the drug. This acts via a similar cellular mechanism of action as described above and achieves erection in 30–60% of patients.

Other intracavernosal agents (unlicensed) include papaverine, phentolamine, a short acting alpha adrenoreceptor blockade, and in combination with aviptadil, a vasoactive intestinal polypeptide licensed in Europe may also be considered [8].

Special Considerations

Testosterone Replacement Therapy

All patients presenting with ED should have their morning (08:00–11:00) testosterone measured, as recent reviews have demonstrated that testosterone replacement improves libido, the response rate to PDE5 inhibitors, and furthermore ED secondary to hypogonadism is potentially reversible with supplementary testosterone.

If the initial assessment of morning testosterone is border-line or low, this should be repeated as a single result may not be accurate due to the pulsatile rhythm of testosterone release. If hypogonadism is found, a referral to Specialist Endocri-nology may be considered as a cause of the hypogonadism should be sought (see Chap. 13). However, treatment for ED can be initiated.

Once a trial period of testosterone therapy has been com-menced, erectile response should be assessed; if erectile sta-tus has improved, testosterone therapy should be continued. If no significant improvement has been observed despite adequate serum testosterone level, combination therapy with PDE5 inhibitors should be started. This combination therapy approach should also be employed in patients with ED who have failed PDE5 inhibitor treatment in whom testosterone levels have not been checked.

Diabetes Mellitus

The prevalence of ED is higher in patients with diabetes [1], similarly, men with diabetes are at higher risk of developing ED. The reported efficacy of PDE5 inhibitors is lower in men with diabetes, making this group of patients more "difficult to treat." This may be because ED, diabetes, and hypogonad-ism often co-exist. Furthermore, diabetes is a risk factor for cardiovascular disease, which in itself is a risk factor for ED, with the underlying etiology most likely involving endothelial dysfunction. This makes patients with ED and diabetes a sub-group of patients where a multiple target approach should be employed; these include long-term adequate glycemic con-trol, assessment, and treatment of concomitant hypogonad-ism and treatment of ED itself.

Patients with diabetes are more prone to infection, making them less desirable candidates for penile implant insertion. Therefore, maximum nonsurgical therapy should be tried before consideration is given to surgical interventions.

Other combination therapies may be considered in selected patients where conservative first- and second-line agents have failed.

Combination Therapy

In patients where monotherapy of oral PDE5 inhibitors or intrac-avernosal injections have failed, a combination therapy approach may be considered [8]; however, one must bear in mind that these combinations are not conventionally recommended regimes and should only be considered in selected patients with careful patient education and counseling prior to initiation of treatment.

Options include combining one oral PDE5 inhibitor with alprostadil injection, or combining alprostadil with papaverine injections due to their different mechanisms of action, or alter-natively combining phentolamine with alprostadil injections.

Once Daily PDE5 Inhibitors

Although the traditional on-demand treatment of ED with PDE5 inhibitors has been demonstrated to be effective, one of the main criticisms has been the "scheduled" nature of sex-ual activity around drug treatment with a lack of spontaneity. Tadalafil has a long half life making this an ideal candidate for a daily dosing regime. Recent studies have demonstrated once daily Tadalafil to be safe, well–tolerated, and most impor-tantly effective in treatment of ED [18], making it a safe alter-native to the current on-demand regime; consequently, sexual activity does not need to be scheduled around tablet taking.

This daily regime has also been shown to be successful in the treatment of ED in diabetic patients in whom ED is somewhat refractory to treatment [19]. There has been no similar study with sildenafil; and with vardenafil, a daily dosing regime was not shown to be superior when compared with the on-demand regime [20]. Currently, the US Food and Drug Administration has approved a daily dosing regime of 2.5 or 5 mg tadalafil.

Key Points

1. PDE5 inhibitors act by inhibiting PDE, which in turn leads to reduced breakdown of intracellular cGMP, leading to reduction in the intracellular concentration of calcium and initiating the process of erection.

2. Careful medical and detailed sexual history enables an accurate diagnosis of ED and establishes a possible underlying cause.
3. ED is associated with cardiovascular disease and hypogonadism. Therefore, patients should be screened for risk factors of cardiovascular diseases and hypogonadism.
4. The rate of response to oral pharmacological agents is improved by effective communication and patient education.
5. Patients should be given the opportunity to trial all PDE5 inhibitors. They can choose their preferred option. The management plan should be tailored to the needs of individual patients.

References

1. Feldman HA, Goldstein I, Hatzichristou DG, Krane RJ, McKinlay JB (1994) Impotence and its medical and psychosocial correlates: results of the Massachusetts male aging study. J Urol 151(1):54–61
2. Andersson KE (2003) Erectile physiological and pathophysiological pathways involved in erectile dysfunction. J Urol 170(2 Pt 2):S6–S13
3. Chiurlia E, D'Amico R, Ratti C, Granata AR, Romagnoli R, Modena MG (2005) Subclinical coronary artery atherosclerosis in patients with erectile dysfunction. J Am Coll Cardiol 46(8):1503–1506
4. Ponholzer A, Temml C, Mock K, Marszalek M, Obermayr R, Madersbacher S (2005) Prevalence and risk factors for erectile dysfunction in 2869 men using a validated questionnaire. Eur Urol 47(1):80–85
5. Vlachopoulos C, Rokkas K, Ioakeimidis N, Stefanadis C (2007) Inflammation, metabolic syndrome, erectile dysfunction, and coronary artery disease: common links. Eur Urol 52(6):1590–1600
6. Montorsi F, Briganti A, Salonia A, Rigatti P, Margonato A, Macchi A et al (2003) Erectile dysfunction prevalence, time of onset and association with risk factors in 300 consecutive patients with acute chest pain and angiographically documented coronary artery disease. Eur Urol 44(3):360–364
7. Montorsi P, Ravagnani PM, Galli S, Rotatori F, Veglia F, Briganti A et al (2006) Association between erectile dysfunction and

coronary artery disease. Role of coronary clinical presentation and extent of coronary vessels involvement: the COBRA trial. Eur Heart J 27(22):2632–2639

8. Hackett G, Kell P, Ralph D, Dean J, Price D, Speakman M et al (2008) British society for sexual medicine guidelines on the management of erectile dysfunction. J Sex Med 5(8):1841–1865

9. Lue TF, Giuliano F, Montorsi F, Rosen RC, Andersson KE, Althof S et al (2004) Summary of the recommendations on sexual dysfunctions in men. J Sex Med 1(1):6–23

10. Giuliano F, Donatucci C, Montorsi F, Auerbach S, Karlin G, Norenberg C et al (2005) Vardenafil is effective and well-tolerated for treating erectile dysfunction in a broad population of men, irrespective of age. BJU Int 95(1):110–116

11. Montorsi F, Verheyden B, Meuleman E, Junemann KP, Moncada I, Valiquette L et al (2004) Long-term safety and tolerability of tadalafil in the treatment of erectile dysfunction. Eur Urol 45(3):339–344

12. Boshier A, Wilton LV, Shakir SA (2004) Evaluation of the safety of sildenafil for male erectile dysfunction: experience gained in general practice use in England in 1999. BJU Int 93(6):796–801

13. Gruenwald I, Shenfeld O, Chen J, Raviv G, Richter S, Cohen A et al (2006) Positive effect of counseling and dose adjustment in patients with erectile dysfunction who failed treatment with sildenafil. Eur Urol 50(1):134–140

14. Ljunggren C, Hedelin H, Salomonsson K, Stroberg P (2008) Giving patients with erectile dysfunction the opportunity to try all three available phosphodiesterase type 5 inhibitors contributes to better long-term treatment compliance. J Sex Med 5(2):469–475

15. Stroberg P, Hedelin H, Ljunggren C (2006) Prescribing all phosphodiesterase 5 inhibitors to a patient with erectile dysfunction – a realistic and feasible option in everyday clinical practice – outcomes of a simple treatment regime. Eur Urol 49(5):900–907

16. British National Formulary. Publisher Pharmaceutical Press; 56 edition (1 Sep 2008). ISBN-13: 978-0853697787

17. The long-term safety of alprostadil (prostaglandin-E1) in patients with erectile dysfunction. The European Alprostadil Study Group (1998). Br J Urol: 82(4):538–543

18. Porst H, Rajfer J, Casabe A, Feldman R, Ralph D, Vieiralves LF et al (2008) Long-term safety and efficacy of tadalafil 5 mg dosed once daily in men with erectile dysfunction. J Sex Med 5(9):2160–2169

19. Hatzichristou D, Gambla M, Rubio-Aurioles E, Buvat J, Brock GB, Spera G et al (2008) Efficacy of tadalafil once daily in men with diabetes mellitus and erectile dysfunction. Diabet Med 25(2):138–146

20. Zumbe J, Porst H, Sommer F, Grohmann W, Beneke M, Ulbrich E (2008) Comparable efficacy of once-daily versus on-demand vardenafil in men with mild-to-moderate erectile dysfunction: findings of the RESTORE study. Eur Urol 54(1):204–210

21. Solomon H, Man JW, Jackson G (2003) Erectile dysfunction and the cardiovascular patient: endothelial dysfunction is the common denominator. Heart 89(3):251–253

Chapter 13
Male Hypogonadism

Aikaterini Theodoraki and Pierre-Marc
Gilles Bouloux

Introduction

Anatomy and Physiology

The testes comprise two main functional cellular units, the interstitial cells and the seminiferous tubules. The interstitial or Leydig cells are found between the seminiferous tubules. Luteinizing hormone (LH) produced from the gonadotroph pituitary cells binds to Leydig cell receptors, stimulating the synthesis and secretion of androgens, predominantly testosterone. Small amounts of androstenedione, dehydroepiandrosterone (DHEA), dihydrotestosterone (DHT), and estradiol are also produced. Most of the circulating estradiol in males is produced in the adipose tissue by aromatization of androgens.

The seminiferous tubules constitute 90% of the testicular volume, and consist of the germ cells and the Sertoli cells. It is the unit where spermatogenesis takes place. Sertoli cells secrete various hormones, such as inhibin B and Mullerian inhibitory factor (MIF). Inhibin B inhibits the secretion of follicle stimulating hormone (FSH), through a negative feedback mechanism from the pituitary, and in early puberty, contributes to the maturation of the gonad. The MIF is

A. Theodoraki (✉)
Endocrinology Department, Royal Free Hospital, Centre for Neuroendocrinology, London, NW3 2QG, UK
e-mail: k_theodoraki@yahoo.gr

I.S. Shergill et al. (eds.), *Medical Therapy in Urology*,
DOI 10.1007/978-1-84882-704-2_13,
© Springer-Verlag London Limited 2010

produced in the male embryo from the eighth week of gestation to suppress female sex organ development during differentiation in utero. FSH binds to Sertoli cell receptors and stimulates spermatogenesis, sperm maturation, and inhibin B production. Intratesticular androgens also promote inhibin B synthesis. Serum inhibin B levels in adults correlate positively with spermatogenesis and can be used as a clinical marker of Sertoli cell function.

Gonadotropin releasing hormone (GnRH) is secreted in pulses from the hypothalamus under the influence of excitatory and inhibitory neurotransmitters and testicular feedback. GnRH regulates the expression of the LH and FSH subunit genes in pituitary gonadotrophs and subsequent LH and FSH secretion. Faster GnRH pulse frequencies promote LH secretion, whereas slower GnRH pulse frequencies favor FSH secretion. Pulsatile GnRH release is essential for gonadotrophin secretion, as exposure to continuous GnRH secretion would lead to downregulation of GnRH receptors and abolish both LH and FSH secretion. Testosterone and other sex steroids inhibit GnRH release from the hypothalamus and LH release from the pituitary. Inhibin B, through a negative feedback loop, inhibits FSH secretion. Other hormone peptides produced in the testes, such as activin and follistatin, also play a role in regulating hypothalamic GnRH secretion [1].

Testosterone has a circadian rhythm with maximum secretion at around 8 am and minimum at 4–9 pm. Only 2–4% of circulating testosterone is free in plasma, the remainder being bound to proteins, mainly albumin (30–50%) and sex hormone binding globulin (SHBG: 45%). Bioavailable testosterone consists of free and albumin-bound testosterone. In the testes, high concentrations of testosterone are essential in the early phases of spermatogenesis. In several target tissues (e.g., prostate, scalp) testosterone is enzymatically converted to DHT by 5α-reductase. DHT is a more potent androgen essential for normal virilization and sexual development. Androgens play a key role in male sexual differentiation during embryogenesis, pubertal male secondary sex characteristics development, male sexual function and behavior, spermatogenesis, and regulation of gonadotropin secretion.

In spermatogenesis, both LH and FSH are required at least at puberty. The whole process takes approximately 72 days followed by another 12–21 days for sperm transport through the epididymis [2].

Classification and Causes of Hypogonadism

Any insult in the hypothalamus–pituitary–gonadal axis (HPG) may result in impaired gonadal function and hypogonadism. Hypogonadism can be classified according to the site involved and the LH, FSH serum levels:

1. Hypogonadotrophic or secondary hypogonadism. It results from inadequate secretion of GnRH or pituitary gonadotrophins. Testosterone is low, and serum LH and FSH are low or inappropriately normal.
2. Hypergonadotrophic or primary hypogonadism. It results from testicular failure. Testosterone is reduced and serum LH and FSH raised.

In both types, the causes may be further subdivided into congenital or acquired and functional or structural (Table 13.1).

The most prevalent functional hypogonadotrophic hypogonadism is seen in aging men, and has been termed "late-onset hypogonadism" (LOH). Drugs such as opiates, glucocorticoids, and cocaine are recognized causes of secondary hypogonadism (Table 13.1). Any structural or infiltrating lesion in the hypothalamic–pituitary region can cause hypogonadotrophic hypogonadism.

Clinical Assessment and Diagnosis

In most cases, male hypogonadism is diagnosed through history, physical examination, and a few basic hormonal assessments [1]. To define the etiology and extent of the HPG axis dysfunction, further tests may be needed. The clinical presentation depends on the age of onset, the severity, and the duration [1, 2]. Hypogonadism is often unrecognized before

TABLE 13.1.   Causes of male hypogonadism.

Hypogonadotrophic hypogonadism	
Congenital	Acquired
• Idiopathic hypogonadotrophic hypogonadism	• Tumors (prolactinomas, craniopharyngiomas)
• Kallmann syndrome	• Infiltrative diseases (hemochromatosis, histiocytosis, sarcoidosis)
• Fertile eunuch syndrome	• Surgery
• Congenital adrenal hypoplasia	• Head trauma
• Associated with multiple pituitary hormone deficiencies	• Radiotherapy
	• Pituitary apoplexy
	• Exercise/weight changes/stress
	• Drugs: anabolic steroids, glucocorticoids, opioids, cocaine, any drug that causes hyperprolactinemia
	• Any acute illness: myocardial infarction, sepsis etc.
	• Chronic illnesses: Crohn's disease, celiac, cystic fibrosis, etc.
	• Hypothyroidism, Cushing's
Hypergonadotrophic hypogonadism	
Congenital	Acquired
• Klinefelter syndrome and other chromosomal disorders	• Orchitis (mumps, HIV)
	• Testicular trauma/torsion
	• Drugs (alkylating agents, sulfasalazine, colchicine, statins, ketoconazole alcohol in excess)
• Androgen synthesis disorders	• Radiotherapy
• Mutations in FSH receptor gene	• Chronic illnesses: chronic renal failure, liver cirrhosis, hemochromatosis
• Cryptorchidism	• Environmental toxins
• Myotonic dystrophy	
• Androgen insensitivity syndromes	

puberty unless it is associated with growth retardation, other endocrine and anatomic abnormalities. When the age of onset is prepubertal, it usually presents with delayed puberty, with the absence of secondary sexual characteristics at an age more than two standard deviations above the population mean for pubertal onset. In that case, testes are small (<5 ml in volume) with a small penis (<5 cm long, <3 cm circumference); there is scanty pubic, axillary, body, and facial hair, central fat distribution, and reduced male musculature may be observed, disproportionately long arms and legs (eunuchoidism, when arm span 1 cm greater than height and lower segment > upper segment, the result of delayed epiphyseal closure), gynecomastia, delayed bone age, and high pitched voice.

In postpubertal hypogonadism, symptoms and signs are due to testosterone deficiency and/or infertility [3, 4]. Progressive decrease in muscle mass with concomitant increase in visceral fat mass, impotence, loss of libido, oligospermia/azoospermia, soft testes with <15 ml volume, gynecomastia, normal male hair distribution, but reduced hair amount, osteoporosis are known sequelae of post-pubertal hypogonadism. With acute onset hypogonadism, menopausal type hot flushes are also described. Other nonspecific symptoms and signs are also associated with hypogonadism, such as decreased energy, motivation, aggressiveness, depressed mood, poor memory and concentration, and normochromic, normocytic anemia.

Recent interest has focused on the prevalence and characteristics of LOH. It is described as a clinical and biochemical syndrome associated with advancing age and characterized by typical symptoms and low serum testosterone levels [5]. The symptoms associated with LOH are those described for post-pubertal onset hypogonadism. For its diagnosis, both clinical features and low serum testosterone are required.

In any case where hypogonadism is suspected, during history taking it is important to ask about developmental defects, e.g., any urinary tract abnormalities or cryptorchidism, the age of onset of puberty, history of any abdominal/genital trauma, testicular torsion, anosmia, drug history, chronic illnesses, family history, and sexual history – erectile function and frequency of intercourse.

The clinical examination should document abnormalities of body hair, muscle mass and fat distribution, possible eunuchoid proportions, and the presence of gynecomastia. Genital examination comprises pubic hair development, phallus and testicular size, and consistency. Normal testes volume is >15 ml with firm consistency. If pituitary disease is suspected, visual fields should be assessed.

Hormone evaluation of testicular function includes the measurement of serum testosterone, SHBG, LH, FSH, and estradiol. Serum testosterone levels vary by 30% during the day, with the peak levels occurring in the early morning. A serum sample obtained around 9 am or between 8 and 11 am is advised [4, 5]. Most of the serum testosterone in bound to SHBG, while the rest (called bioavailable testosterone) is bound to albumin and 2–4% is unbound (free testosterone). Non-SHBG-bound testosterone comprises the biologically active component that is readily available in the tissues [4].

SHBG levels may be affected by a variety of conditions, thereby influencing the total testosterone concentration. SHBG may be low in obesity, nephrotic syndrome, acromegaly, hypothyroidism, following administration of glucocorticoids, anabolic steroids, and progesterone. In contrast, SHBG levels are increased with aging, liver cirrhosis, growth hormone deficiency, hyperthyroidism, and following administration of estrogens [2, 6]. When measuring serum gonadotropins, it is important to note that LH and FSH are secreted in short pulses, with FSH having a longer half-life, thus being a more accurate indicator in a single measurement [1]. If the testosterone level measured is low, it should be repeated along with LH and FSH values. Estradiol/estrone in men results largely from peripheral aromatization of testosterone and androstenedione in adipose tissue. A small amount of estradiol is also secreted by Leydig cells. Causes of raised estrogens in men are liver disease, obesity, hyperthyroidism, androgen resistance syndromes, antiandrogen therapy, primary testicular failure, and tumors that produce estrogens or human chorionic gonadotropin (hCG), such as adrenal and testicular tumors, respectively. In secondary hypogonadism, thyroid function tests and serum prolactin levels are also useful, since both hypothyroidism and hyperprolactinemia are recognized causes of hypogonadotrophic hypogonadism [7].

After the initial hormonal evaluation, specific investigations depending on the suspected cause of hypogonadism may be requested, such as karyotype testing, serum iron studies, MRI pituitary, etc. Dynamic endocrine testing may be used to assess the hypothalamo-pituitary testicular axis further [1]. The interpretation of these tests can be difficult as the ranges of response are poorly defined, thus they are not used in everyday endocrine practice.

If androgen replacement therapy is considered, it is important to measure prostate-specific antigen (PSA) levels, lipid profile, full blood count (hemoglobin and hematocrit) and liver function tests prior to initiating any replacement therapy.

Medical Therapies in Male Hypogonadism

The treatment of male hypogonadism relies largely on whether fertility is desired and on the level of the lesion on the HPG axis. In hypogonadotrophic (secondary) hypogonadism when fertility is the goal of treatment, pulsatile GnRH therapy using a subcutaneous infusion pump and syringe may be used to induce gonadotrophin secretion and hence sperm production in suprapituitary lesions. The pump administers boluses of GnRH every 2 h and the dose should be titrated to achieve normal LH, FSH, and testosterone levels [2, 6].

Alternatively, exogenous gonadotropins can be administered subcutaneously or intramuscularly to induce spermatogenesis when fertility is desired in hypogonadotrophic hypogonadism caused either by hypothalamic or pituitary disease [2, 6]. Human chorionic gonadotrophin (hCG) due to its structural homology to LH is used as a substitute to LH to stimulate Leydig cells to synthesis and secretion of testosterone. Both urinary and recombinant hCG preparations are available. FSH can be administered in the form of human menopausal gonadotrophins (hMG) or recombinant FSH [8]. Therapy is typically initiated with hCG alone and the dose is titrated based on trough testosterone levels and testicular growth.

In the majority of patients with larger testes at baseline (>5 ml), spermatogenesis may initiate with hCG alone due to residual FSH secretion. The main side-effect of exogenous gonadotropins is gynecomastia. In terms of monitoring the response, once testes are >8 ml in size, semen analysis should be performed at regular intervals. Sperm appears in the ejaculate in up to 90% cases, though often not to normal counts. Pregnancy can be achieved normally or with the help of an assisted reproductive technique, although it is a curious observation that males may be fertile with counts as low as 1 million/ml [6].

However, the mainstay of treatment of male hypogonadism is androgen-replacement therapy in the form of testosterone. Multiple delivery systems are currently available such as oral preparations, buccal, transdermal (patches or gels), intramuscular injections, and pellets (Table 13.2).

The benefits of testosterone replacement therapy depend on the age of the male patient [2, 4, 6]. Testosterone can restore libido, erectile function, and the secondary male sexual characteristics inducing virilization in the young male. It can result in improvement in mood, energy levels, and well-being. Testosterone replacement also has been shown to change the body composition causing an increase in lean body mass and a reduction in fat mass. Testosterone inhibits bone resorption and it is known to improve bone mineral density in hypogonadal males – however, the effects on fracture risk are not known. There is also a dose-dependent increase in hemoglobin levels with testosterone administration, greater in older men. Prospective population studies have also shown an association between low testosterone levels and an increased risk for type 2 diabetes, the metabolic syndrome, and reduced survival, especially due to cardiovascular or respiratory mortality [6, 9]. It is not known, however, if testosterone replacement therapy reduces the risk for type 2 diabetes or the metabolic syndrome or improves life expectancy.

Testosterone is contraindicated in breast or prostate malignancy, as these are hormone-dependent cancers and may be stimulated to grow with testosterone therapy. It is also contraindicated where there is suspicion of prostate cancer (e.g. with palpable prostate nodules/induration or raised PSA) without prior urological evaluation, in patients with severe lower urinary tract symptoms suggestive of benhign prostatic hyperplasia (BPH) (international prostate symptom score >19), in erythrocytosis (hematocrit >50%), in untreated obstructive sleep apnoea, or in unstable severe congestive heart failure [3, 4].

Despite the benefits of testosterone replacement in hypogonadal males, adverse effects are recognized and should be explained to the patient and sought in clinic visits. Erythrocytosis is a dose-dependent treatment side-effect that occurs mainly in older males. It is more frequently observed with injectable testosterone preparations (in up to 44% of patients) than with transdermal administration (in 3–18% patients). If it occurs, dose reduction, withholding of testosterone treatment, therapeutic phlebotomy, or blood donation can be considered [3]. In any hypogonadal male on testosterone replacement, hematocrit checks prior to each clinic visit are recommended.

In terms of BPH, prostate volume increases during testosterone therapy of hypogonadal males, but only to a volume expected of a normal control male. This increase, however, does not seem to correlate with worsening of urinary symptoms. Testosterone replacement may unmask previously clinically unrecognized prostate cancer. Monitoring with digital rectal examination (DRE) and PSA values in patients >45 years and the threshold for prostate biopsy if DRE is abnormal or if PSA rises should be low. It is under debate if testosterone could be administered in patients treated from prostate cancer [10].

Hepatotoxic effects and neoplasia were previously observed with 17α-methyl-testosterone and other substitute compounds. These oral preparations are no longer recommended [3]. Current oral preparations are oil soluble (testosterone undecanoate), absorbed by the intestinal lymphatics, and bypass the liver first-pass metabolism.

Fears for cardiovascular risk with testosterone therapy do not seem substantiated since existing evidence suggests a neutral or possible beneficial effect [3]. With supra-physiological testosterone doses, a reduction in HDL cholesterol has been observed. With physiological testosterone doses, most studies show a neutral effect on serum lipids.

TABLE 13.2.   Medical therapy of male hypogonadism.

Testosterone preparations				
Name	Mode of action	Dose	Side-effects	Contraindications
Oral testosterone undecanoate	Binds to testosterone receptors in androgen-dependent tissues	120–160 mg daily for 2–3 weeks, then 40–120 mg daily in 2–3 divided doses, with meals	Erythrocytosis, sleep apnoea, acne, seborrhoea, gynecomastia, edema, male pattern baldness, hypertension, possibly prostatic hyperplasia and unmasking prostate cancer; precocious sexual development and premature closure of epiphyses in pre-pubertal males; suppression of spermatogenesis in men	Prostate or breast cancer, erythrocytosis, sleep apnoea, severe heart failure, severe prostatic hyperplasia symptoms
Testosterone mucoadhesive buccal tablets	As above	30 mg every 12 h	As above Also gum-related adverse event in 16% patients; taste alterations	As above
Testosterone undecanoate intramuscular injection	As above	1 g every 10–14 weeks second dose may be given after 6 weeks for rapid plasma levels	As with oral testosterone undecanoate	As above

Testosterone esters: enanthate and propionate, intramuscular injections	As above	Dose depends on the ester/esters used: testosterone enanthate 250 mg every 2–3 weeks initially, maintenance 3–6 weekly Testosterone propionate 50 mg 2–3 times weekly Testosterone esters mixture 1 mL every 2–3 weeks depending on the dose	As above; also due to variations in serum testosterone levels achieved possible "roller coaster" effect with androgen deficiency symptoms occurring before next injection	As above
Testosterone pellets; implanted SC using trocar	As above	100 or 200 mg pellets available; 4–6 implanted every 4–6 months	As with oral testosterone undecanoate; pellets may extrude spontaneously; risk of local skin infections	As above
Transdermal testosterone patches	As above	2.5 or 5 mg/24 h	As with oral testosterone undecanoate Also skin reactions (erythema, pruritus, burn-like lesions in up to 66% of patients)	As above

(continued)

TABLE 13.2.   (continued)

Testosterone preparations

Name	Mode of action	Dose	Side-effects	Contraindications
Transdermal testosterone gel	As above	50 mg/sachet or 10 mg/metered application; 50–80 mg applied o.d.	As with oral testosterone undecanoate Also skin irritation and allergic reactions in ≈ 5% patients Risk of testosterone transfer by skin contact to female partner or child	As above

Drugs when fertility is the aim of treatment in male hypogonadotrophic hypogonadism

Name	Mode of action	Dose	Side-effects	Contraindications
Gonadotropin releasing hormone (GnRH)	Stimulates the synthesis and secretion of LH and FSH from the pituitary gonadotrophs	25–600 ng/kg administered with a sc pump every 90–120 min	Nausea, headache, abdominal pain; hypersensitivity reaction on large doses repeated administration; irritation at injection sites	Caution in pituitary adenoma
Human chorionic gonadotropin – urine derived or recombinant (hCG)	Stimulates the synthesis and secretion of testosterone	1,000–2,000 IU IM 2–3/week	Edema, headache, tiredness, gynecomastia	Androgen-dependent tumors; tumors of hypothalamus and pituitary
Recombinant human follicle stimulation hormone (rFSH)	Induces spermatogenesis	75–150 IU IM ×3/week	Headache, gastrointestinal symptoms, gynecomastia, fever, acne	Tumors of the hypothalamus, pituitary, testes, or prostate

Testosterone therapy seems to be associated with exacerbation or development of sleep apnoea, especially in men treated with high doses of intramuscular testosterone and who have other risk factors for sleep apnoea. It seems that testosterone contributes to sleep disordered breathing by central mechanisms, since the upper airway dimensions do not alter with testosterone therapy [3].

Skin reaction such as erythema and pruritus are common with transdermal testosterone preparations – up to 66% with patches and 5% with gels. Acne, oily skin, breast tenderness, and occasionally gynecomastia may be observed especially in young individuals [3, 8].

Testosterone is known to cause sodium and water retention; however, it is rarely of clinical significance.

Exogenous testosterone as a sex steroid suppresses the production of gonadotropins; hence, it commonly causes testicular atrophy and infertility. These effects are usually reversible.

Monitoring for the safety and efficacy of testosterone treatment is recommended (Table 13.3). The efficacy of treatment correlates with serum testosterone levels. Therapy should aim to raise serum testosterone levels to the mid-normal range. When to measure testosterone levels depends on the delivery system [4]. With injectable testosterone preparations, levels can be measured midway between injections, with transdermal patches 3–12 h after application of the patch, with buccal testosterone bioadhesive tablet levels can be assessed immediately before or after application of fresh system. With the transdermal gel, testosterone level can be measured any time after the patient has been on treatment for at least 1 week; with oral testosterone undecanoate 3–5 h after ingestion; with injectable testosterone undecanoate serum testosterone level can be measured just prior to each subsequent injection. If levels are low, then adjustment of the dose administered (or the interval between injections) is advised. Clinic reviews are advised 2–3 months after testosterone initiation, then in 6 months and yearly. With transdermal preparations, the testosterone levels achieved often are in the low/normal range. If androgen deficiency symptoms are still present, consider changing to injectable testosterone.

TABLE 13.3.   Recommendations for monitoring testosterone replacement therapy.

Baseline	• Measure baseline testosterone, Hct/hemoglobin, and PSA
	• Ask for urinary voiding symptoms or use questionnaire, such as the IPSS
	• Perform DRE
	• If PSA is >4 ng/ml or DRE is abnormal, refer for prostate biopsy
	• Ask for symptoms of sleep apnoea
	• If history of fragility fractures or very low testosterone levels assess bone mineral density
Follow up	• Assess the patients in 3 months for efficacy of treatment and potential side-effects
	• Adjust dose/interval of testosterone administration if suboptimal response
	• Measure testosterone, PSA, and Hct in 3 months, 6 months, and if no concern annually thereafter
	• If history of osteoporosis or fragility fractures assess bone mineral density every 2 years
	• Perform DRE in every visit in patients >45 years old
	• If PSA is > 4.0 ng/ml or if there is an increase in serum PSA >1.4 ng/ml within any 12-month period of testosterone treatment or a PSA velocity of >0.4 ng/ml/year using the PSA level after 6 months of testosterone administration as the reference (only applicable if PSA data are available for a period exceeding 2 year) or if a prostatic abnormality is detected on DRE, then ask for urology review

Notes:
Hct: Hematocrit
PSA: Prostate Specific Antigen
IPSS: International Prostate Symptom Score
DRE: Digital Rectal Examination

Key points

1. Male Hypogonadism is the failure of testes to produce adequate amount of testosterone, spermatozoa, or both. It can be classified into hypogonadotrophic or secondary hypogonadism and hypergonadotrophic or primary hypogonadism.
2. History, clinical examination, and a few hormonal assessments are used to differentiate between the main types

of hypogonadism. More specific tests may be required to identify the cause further.

3. Testosterone replacement therapy has multiple benefits for the hypogonadal male. There are multiple formulations for testosterone administration and an individualized approach is needed according to the patient.

4. Monitoring for the safety and efficacy of testosterone with regular testosterone serum levels, hematocrit, PSA, and clinical assessment including DRE is advised.

5. If fertility is the aim of treatment in hypogonadotrophic hypogonadism, GnRH pulse therapy or exogenous gonadotropins may be given.

References

1. Isidori AM, Giannetta E, Lenzi A (2008) Male hypogonadism. Pituitary 11:171–180
2. Turner HE, Wass JAH (2002) Oxford Handbook of Endocrinology and Diabetes. Oxford University Press 417–443
3. Rhoden EL, Morgentaler A (2004) Risks of testosterone replacement therapy and recommendations for monitoring. New Engl J Med 350:482–492
4. Bhasin S, Cunningham GR, Hayes FJ, et al. (2006) Testosterone therapy in adult men with androgen deficiency syndromes: an endocrine society clinical practice guideline. J Clin Endocrinol Metab 91:1995–2010
5. Nieschlag E, Swerdloff R, Behre HM et al. (2006) Investigation, treatment and monitoring of late-onset hypogonadism in males: ISA, ISSAM and EAU recommendations. Journal of Andrology 27(2):135–137
6. Beg S, Al-Khoury L, Cunningham GR (2008) Testosterone replacement in men. Current Opinion in Endocrinology, Diabetes and Obesity 15:364–370
7. Traish AM, Goldstein I, Kim NN (2007) Testosterone and erectile function: from basic research to a new clinical paradigm for managing men with androgen insufficiency and erectile dysfunction. European Urology 54–70
8. British National Formulary 56 (2008) Male sex hormones and antagonists. Hypothalamic and anterior pituitary hormones. 399–404

9. Laughlin GA, Barrett-Connor E, Bergstrom J (2008) Low serum testosterone and mortality in older men. J Clin Endocrinol Metab 93:68–75

10. Dobs AS, Morgentaler A (2008) Does testosterone therapy increase the risk of prostate cancer? Endcor Pract 14(7):904–911

Chapter 14
Renal Transplantation

Behdad Afzali, Kerem B. Atalar, Refik Gökmen and
David J.A. Goldsmith

Introduction

Advances in vascular surgery permitted the first successful
renal transplant between identical twins by Joseph Murray's
group at the Peter Bent Brigham Hospital in Boston in 1954.
This procedure was carried out without any immunosuppressive medication as both donor and recipient carried the
same histocompatibility genes, minimizing immunological
responses to the transplant. Over 50 years later, advances in
tissue typing and immunosuppression have made transplantation of kidneys between genetically disparate (allogeneic)
individuals the treatment of choice for surgically fit patients
with end-stage renal failure. Patients with renal allografts
have considerably better morbidity and mortality than those
on hemodialysis (although this observation is confounded by
the self-selection of patients with better functional status to
undergo transplantation, it remains true) and substantially
more independence and better quality of life.

Nevertheless, despite the introduction of new and expensive
immunosuppressive agents, improvements in allograft lifespan

D. J. A. Goldsmith (✉)
MRC Centre for Transplantation, Department of Nephrology and Transplantation, 6th Floor, Borough Wing, Guy's Hospital, London SE1 9RT.
e-mail: david.goldsmith@gstt.nhs.uk

I.S. Shergill et al. (eds.), *Medical Therapy in Urology,*   197
DOI 10.1007/978-1-84882-704-2_14,
© Springer-Verlag London Limited 2010

have lagged behind those in 1-year survival (now routinely >90%). The commonest cause of long-term graft loss remains death with a functioning graft, from a marked excess of cardiovascular mortality in allograft recipients. This is closely followed by chronic allograft injury (CAI), the term given to the development of fibrotic processes leading to progressive allograft dysfunction. CAI can be the end result of a number of different pathologies, including chronic rejection, hypertension, and chronic calcineurin inhibitor toxicity. The success of transplantation is further limited by the consequences of long-term immunosuppression, namely an excess of malignancy and infectious diseases.

It is the purpose of this chapter to review the medical management of patients with renal allografts, concentrating in particular on immunosuppression, cardiovascular risk reduction, and transplant surveillance.

Principles and History of Anti-Rejection Therapies

In the early 1960s, the introduction of immunosuppressant drugs for the prevention of transplant rejection heralded the beginning of an era of intensive research into optimal strategies for immunomodulation. A wide range of treatment modalities have since been developed, but the therapeutic aims of each of these can be simplified to a set of broad principles. Essentially, immunomodulation should inhibit the immune response to the graft such that it is no longer at risk of rejection, while at the same time, maintaining the recipient's capability to adequately combat threats, such as infection and neoplasia. These goals must be balanced with general therapeutic principles such as limiting the side-effects of drugs and allowing patients to maintain an acceptable quality of life. The immunomodulatory strategies that have been investigated in pursuit of these objectives can be loosely grouped into two major approaches: immunosuppression and tolerance induction. To date, immunosuppression has enjoyed remarkable clinical success in improving the outcome of transplantation, while tolerance induction remains a focus of ongoing research.

Immunomodulatory Modalities, Protocols, and Clinical Trials

The various classes of immunomodulatory therapies include chemical drugs, protein-based therapeutics (that may utilize antibodies or antibody fragments), and other techniques such as extracorporeal column-based antibody depletion strategies. Table 14.1 details the most important and frequently encountered examples of these treatments, along with their mechanism of action, important associated risks, and notes on the usage of each.

In modern clinical practice, multiple therapeutic modalities are commonly used in combination to minimize the dosage of individual agents and maximize effectiveness in the prevention of rejection.

Initially, a specific course of treatment is given during the perioperative period to induce effective immunosuppression at the time of transplantation when immunological reactivity is at its peak. This induction regimen usually includes protein therapy (such as anti-CD25 antibody), as well as chemical drugs. Alongside this, lifelong maintenance immunosuppression is commenced, although this is generally reduced and modified over time as the risk of acute rejection diminishes. Episodes of acute rejection are identified and treated as they occur. Owing to expansions in available pharmaceuticals, there is now considerable inter-center variation in transplant immunosuppression protocols. Nevertheless, the majority of centers maintain patients in the long term with a combination of low-dose steroids and two steroid sparing agents, usually a calcineurin inhibitor and an anti-proliferative agent.

Most clinical trials in transplantation report a composite endpoint that comprises patient survival, graft survival, and acute rejection incidence, but comparing trials to determine the best therapeutic regimen has become exceedingly difficult because of the large number of potential drug combinations and complex protocols.

Acute Rejection

For most patients, episodes of acute rejection are treated successfully with short courses of high-dose corticosteroids,

TABLE 14.1.   Medical therapy in renal transplantation.

Name	Mode of action	Dose	Side-effects	Notes
Calcineurin inhibitors Cyclosporine Tacrolimus	Inhibit production of IL-2 and other cytokines, resulting in impaired T cell activation and proliferation		Direct nephrotoxicity (cyclosporine > tacrolimus), hypertension, hyperlipidemia (cyclosporine > tacrolimus), neurotoxicity (tacrolimus)	Serum drug levels require monitoring. Tacrolimus thought to be more potent than cyclosporine and used in preference to cyclosporine in sensitized patients and in combined kidney-pancreas transplantation. Cyclosporine introduced clinically in early 1980s, tacrolimus in mid-1990s. Currently used widely.
mTOR inhibitors Sirolimus Everolimus	Block lymphocyte cell-cycle activity, thereby inhibiting lymphocyte proliferation		Poor wound healing, oral ulceration, hyperlipidemia, thrombocytopenia, post-transplant diabetes mellitus	Introduced in late-1990s, current role unclear from evidence. Less nephrotoxicity than CNIs. Investigated as potential monotherapeutic agent. May be a more favorable drug for tolerance inducing strategies
Anti-proliferatives Azathioprine Mycophenolate mofetil (MMF)	both inhibit purine synthesis; azathioprine interferes with DNA synthesis; both result in impaired lymphocyte proliferation; MMF has additional anti-B cell activity		Bone marrow suppression, GI disturbance (MMF especially), leukopenia, hepatocellular injury (azathioprine), trophic skin changes, and malignancies (especially azathioprine)	Azathioprine revolutionized transplantation in 1960s; now used far less frequently – mycophenolate preferred due to superior side-effect

Corticosteroids Prednisolone Methyl- prednisolone	Bind cytosolic glucocorticoid receptor and thereby up/down-regulate expression of multiple genes in multiple cell types. Potent immunosuppressants at high dose	Very wide-ranging; examples include post-transplant diabetes mellitus, hypertension, hyperlipidemia, peptic ulceration, psychosis, pancreatitis, osteoporosis	Commonly used as part of induction and early immunosuppression protocols. Effective in treatment episodes of acute rejection episodes
Other Deoxyspergua- line (DSG) Tresperimus	Inhibits T cell proliferation and cytokine production	Leukopenia	Still experimental; rarely used in regular clinical practice outside of Japan and Far East
Anti-IL2 Receptor antibodies Basiliximab Daclizumab	Block CD25 (IL-2 receptor) on T cells, inhibiting the proliferation of these cells and reducing their contribution to rejection	Long-term risks not yet defined	Introduced in 2000s; now commonly used as part of immunosuppression induction regimen. Less risk of opportunistic infections than drugs such as CNIs and corticosteroids
Polyclonal anti-T cell antibodies Anti-thymocyte globulin (ATG)	Lymphocyte depletion by binding of multiple epitopes found on T cells	Increased infection rate post-transplant, increased incidence of malignancy (particularly associated with post-transplant lymphoproliferative disease, PTLD), infusion-related symptoms	Commonly used as induction agent (particularly in the US); may be used as treatment for acute rejection
Monoclonal anti-T cell antibodies Muromonab (OKT3)	Binds a T cell receptor component, inhibiting T cell activation and proliferation M	Cytokine release syndrome, CMV infection	The first monoclonal antibody licensed for use in transplantation; less commonly used now

(continued)

TABLE 14.1.   (continued)

Name	Mode of action	Dose	Side-effects	Notes
Monoclonal anti-B cell antibodies Rituximab	Depletion of B cells by binding to CD20, which results in B cell lysis, reducing B cell contribution to antibody production and as well as antigen presentation		Infusion-related symptoms	May be used as rescue therapy during episodes of antibody-mediated acute rejection or for resistant cell-mediated rejection
Monoclonal anti-lymphocyte antibodies Alemtuzumab (Campath-1)	Targets CD52, a surface protein found on mature lymphocytes, resulting in profound lymphocyte depletion		Infusion-related symptoms; long-term risks unknown at present	Experimental; originally introduced as treatment for chronic lymphocytic leukemia and T cell lymphoma; now being investigated for role in tolerance induction
CTLA4-Ig fusion proteins Abatacept Belatacept	Inhibits T cell activation by binding a key costimulatory surface molecule found on antigen-presenting cells		Infusion-related symptoms; long-term risks unknown	Experimental; noninferiority to cyclosporine in acute rejection incidence has been demonstrated; further trials ongoing
Immunoad-sorption	Removal of preformed antibodies from recipient serum by column-based approach		Relatively recent introduction; used prior to ABO blood group incompatible transplantation and in patients who are highly sensitized to HLA antigens	

which are sometimes supplemented with protein therapies such as rituximab and ATG. However, these events remain an important determinant of long-term graft survival, even when treated. Advances in immunosuppression have progressively reduced the incidence of acute rejection, but it is still a significant problem in the long term. Most patients can expect to have at least one episode of acute rejection in the first 6 months post-transplantation.

Adverse Effects of Immunosuppression

A number of important drug-specific side-effects have fuelled the hunt for improved immunosuppressive agents and regimens, and are worth mentioning here.

The desire to withdraw steroid therapy due to their wide-ranging undesirable effects (particularly metabolic – hypertension, dyslipidemia, impaired glucose tolerance; osteopenia, obesity, and dermal atrophy) has resulted in the incorporation into most protocols of a phased reduction in steroid therapy. Some even omit steroid treatment altogether, while others gradually taper dosage until withdrawal has been completed.

The sustained use of the calcineurin inhibitors cyclosporine and tacrolimus has also been targeted because of their ability to contribute to renal dysfunction through direct nephrotoxicity and by adversely affecting risk factors that may accelerate cardiovascular disease (hypertension, dyslipidemia, impaired glucose tolerance), and cosmetic-functional factors (hirsutes, tremor, GI disturbance). Again, this has led to protocols that either taper therapy to specific target levels (both drugs require continuous therapeutic drug monitoring of plasma levels) or omit calcineurin inhibitors altogether. Finally, the anti-proliferative drug mycophenolate has replaced azathioprine for new transplant recipients on account of its greater efficacy in preventing acute rejection and superior side-effect profile.

The most important general side-effects of immunosuppression are the development of neoplasia and an increased risk of infection. For these reasons, it is desirable to limit the extent of all immunosuppressive therapies, and it is this, in particular, that has inspired the search for novel strategies of tolerance induction.

An ideal tolerance induction protocol would involve a short, safe treatment that reliably promotes graft acceptance by the recipient and allows graft function to be maintained indefinitely in the absence of immunosuppression, without causing any short- or long-term undesirable effects. Multiple reports of successful therapeutic regimens in animal models, combined with the identification of a tiny minority of nonimmunosuppressed renal transplant recipients that do not reject their graft, has encouraged research in this field. However, as yet, a clinically viable technique for tolerance induction has not been described.

Infections

As potent immunosuppressive medications have dramatically reduced the incidence of rejection, infections have become a leading cause of morbidity and mortality among renal transplant recipients. It is important to note that infections can be both more severe and more difficult to recognize in patients taking immunosuppressive therapy than in those with a normal immune system.

Malignancy

In parallel with these infectious complications, there is also a significantly increased incidence of many cancers among renal transplant recipients when compared with dialysis patients and the general population. This increase in incidence applies particularly to malignancies of the skin, lymphoid tissue, and urogenital tract. The total burden of immunosuppressive therapy seems to be the most important risk factor, rather than the use of individual immunosuppressive agents. According to one study, the risk of malignancy after 20 years of immunosuppressive therapy may be as high as 40%. Therefore, the most important measure to prevent cancers is to minimize excessive immunosuppression whenever possible, requiring clinicians to judge the balance between the risks of over- and under-immunosuppression in each individual case.

Renal transplant recipients should be encouraged to take up cancer screening strategies as recommended for the general population, such as mammography, colonoscopy, or cervical cytology. In addition, they should be advised to minimize the risk of skin cancers by minimizing exposure to ultraviolet radiation and using appropriate protection (at least factor 50 sunblock). Particularly in areas with a high risk of skin malignancies, and in those transplant recipients with a long history of immunosuppression, monitoring for premalignant skin lesions should be routine in the transplant clinic.

Cardiovascular Disease

The commonest cause of death in renal allograft recipients remains an excess of cardiovascular mortality (death with a functioning graft). While some of this excess disease burden can be explained by risk factors related to chronic kidney disease pretransplantation such as diabetes, hypertension, anemia, calcium-phosphate imbalance, and chronic inflammation, the *de novo* development of cardiovascular risk factors pots-engraftment also plays a substantial role in imparting cardiovascular risk.

Hypertension and dyslipidemia post-transplantation are almost universal in the renal allograft population, as a result of both local (e.g., renal transplant artery stenosis and poor allograft function) and systemic (notably the effects of immunosuppressive agents such as CNIs and corticosteroids) factors. By the same token, new onset diabetes mellitus (which in some series affects up to 30% of subjects, largely the result of immunosuppressive drugs) and post-transplant anemia, significantly increase the cardiovascular risk. As a result, an important part of the management of the renal transplant recipient is medical cardiovascular risk reduction.

Diabetes

A significant proportion of renal transplant recipients have pre-existing diabetes, reflecting the fact that diabetes mellitus is the leading cause of end-stage renal disease in the developed world. In addition, up to 25% of transplant recipients develop new-onset diabetes after transplantation, with obesity,

Afro-Caribbean and South Asian ethnicity, and use of gluco-corticoids and tacrolimus being particular risk factors. Both pre-existing and new onset diabetes are associated with poor outcomes, both in terms of long-term allograft survival and cardiovascular complications.

Transplant recipients must therefore be screened for the development of diabetes and treated according to established standards in the nontransplant population. Minimization of glucocorticoid therapy and reduction of the tacrolimus dose may also be appropriate. Patients with combined kidney-pancreas transplants are screened with particular diligence for the development of diabetes as elevated blood sugars often indicate poor pancreatic health.

Bone Disease

Although transplantation can ameliorate, or at least halt the progression of the renal bone disease seen in dialysis patients, bone disease continues to be a significant problem following transplantation. Osteoporosis is common, largely due to glucocorticoid therapy; the incidence of avascular necrosis has declined as lower cumulative doses are used. Hyperparathyroidism is common after transplantation, and if caused by suboptimal renal function, ongoing treatment with vitamin D analogs may be indicated. Calcium-sensing receptor drugs (e.g., Cinacalcet) are being used more frequently now.

Hyperuricemia and Gout

Gout is common after renal transplantation, and seems to be particularly associated with cyclosporine therapy. Nonsteroidal anti-inflammatory agents are a potential concern in renal transplant recipients, and many centers would advocate avoiding their use altogether. Allopurinol must also be avoided (or used with great care and at lower dosage) in patients treated with azathioprine as the interaction between these two agents can cause profound marrow suppression. It is worth remembering that losartan has a mild uricosuric effect.

Anemia

Anemia is common following transplantation, largely owing to suboptimal allograft function and the use of medications such as azathioprine, Mycophenolate mofetil (MMF), or ACE inhibitors, which may impair erythropoiesis. Iron deficiency (absolute, or functional) is common. Iron supplementation, followed if needed by erythropoiesis-stimulating agents (ESAs) such a recombinant erythropoietin is therefore common in the post-transplant setting. Although no prospective trial data are available to guide the treatment of post-transplant anemia, it seems reasonable to manage anemia in transplant recipients in a manner similar to that used in other chronic kidney disease patients. Anemia treatment thresholds are Hb<10.5 g/dL and treatment should aim to achieve Hb levels in the range 10.5–12.5 g/dL.

Key Points

1. Transplantation of the kidney is almost always successful in 2009, primarily due to the adjuvant use of medical therapies to present subsequent rejection.
2. Current immunosuppressive modalities have significantly reduced the likelihood of transplant loss from acute rejection – routine transplant survival in most centers is now greater than 90% by the end of the first postoperative year.
3. Complications of long-term broad-spectrum immunosuppression still carry significant morbidity and mortality and necessitate stringent post-transplant surveillance and the reduction of long-term risk.
4. Medical management of complications resulting from the drugs used for immune suppression (e.g. infection, skin changes, diabetes) is key to successful long-term outcomes.
5. The induction of a state of immunological tolerance to transplanted organs without the requirement for pharmacological immunosuppression with retention of the capacity to respond to infectious agents remains the theoretical long-term goal of the transplant team.

Further Reading

1. Anemia after renal transplantation. Afzali B, Al-Khoury S, Shah N, Mikhail A, Covic A, Goldsmith D. Am J Kidney Dis 2006; 48: 519–536.
2. Coronary artery disease in uremia: aetiology, diagnosis and therapy. Civic A, Goldsmith DJ. Kidney Int 2001; 60: 2059–2078.
3. What we CAN do about chronic allograft nephropathy: role of immunosuppressive modulations. Kidney Int 2005; 68: 2429–2443.

Chapter 15
Analgesia for Urological Procedures

Aza A. Mohammed, Rose McRobert, and Brian Little

Introduction

Pain is defined (according to the WHO) as "an unpleasant sensory and emotional experience associated with actual or potential tissue damage, or described in terms of such damage" [1].

The urinary tract is mainly under the control of the autonomic nervous system. Preganglionic sympathetic fibers to the kidneys arise from T8-L1 spinal segments. These converge into the coeliac and aorto-cortical ganglia and then give rise to postganglionic fibers to supply the kidneys. Parasympathetic supply to the kidneys is via the vagus nerve. Preganglionic sympathetic fibers to the ureters originate from T10-L2 spinal segments. These converge into the aorticorenal and superior and inferior hypogastric plexuses. Postganglionic fibers arise from these plexuses to supply the ureters. Parasympathetic input to the ureters is mainly via the S2-4 segments. Somatic pain fibers travel with the sympathetic fibers and therefore patients with renal or ureteric stones manifest with pain referring to the somatic distribution of T10-L2. Sympathetic supply to the bladder originates from T11-L2 segments which travel through the superior hypogastric plexus and supply the bladder through the right and left hypogastric nerves. The sympathetic

A. A. Mohammed (✉)
Department of Urology, The Ayr Hospital, Ayr, KA6 6DX, UK
e-mail: aza_bamerny@yahoo.com

I.S. Shergill et al. (eds.), *Medical Therapy in Urology*,
DOI 10.1007/978-1-84882-704-2_15,
© Springer-Verlag London Limited 2010

system is inhibitory to the detrusor muscle and maintains the tone of the bladder neck. The parasympathetic nerve supply originates from the spinal segments S2-4 to form the pelvic parasympathetic plexus. These are excitatory to the detrusor muscle and inhibitory to the bladder neck. The penis is mainly supplied by the dorsal nerve of the penis, which is a branch of the pudendal nerve (S2-4). These nerves pass underneath the inferior margin of the pubic arch and run within the subpubic space and through the suspensory ligament to reach the inner surface of the Buck's fascia accompanied by the dorsal artery of the penis. The scrotum is innervated anteriorly by the ilio-inguinal and iliohypogastric nerves (L1-2) and posteriorly by the perineal branches of the pudendal nerve (S2-4).

Painful stimuli are carried from the peripheral nerves through the spinal cord into the precentral gyrus of the cerebral cortex via ordered neuronal pathways. The cell bodies of the first-order neurons lie in the dorsal horn and synapse with the second-order neurons. The second-order axons cross the midline and travel via the spinothalamic tract to reach the thalamus. In the thalamus, the second-order neurons synapse with third-order neurons, which project through the internal capsule and corona and then radiate into the sensory cerebral cortex.

Pain usually results from stimulation of the sensory peripheral nerve endings. These are high-threshold nerves which could either be nonmyelinated slow-conducting C fibers (producing dull pain) or myelinated rapidly-conducting A-fibers (producing sharp pain). Tissue injury or ischemia is accompanied by the local release of various chemical substances. These act on the nerve endings causing direct stimulation or increase the sensitivity of these nerve endings to various other stimuli. These chemicals include vanilloids (such as capsaicin), kinines (such as bradykinines), prostaglandins, cations (H^+, K^+), serotinine, histamine and substance P.

Medical Therapies used in Urological Analgesia

The common analgesics used in urological practice are summarised in Table 15.1 and a discussion of their clinical use in procedures is now presented.

Spinal Anesthesia

This provides rapid and complete sensorimotor block below the level of the umbilicus (T10) for 2–3 h. Thus it facilitates surgery without general anesthesia.

The procedure is performed under strict aseptic technique with intravenous access and monitoring. The patient is placed in the sitting or lateral position, with hips and spine flexed. The landmark is a line joining the iliac crests across the spinous process of L4. After infiltration with local anesthesia, an introducer is inserted perpendicular to the skin at the L3/4 interspace and is used to progress through skin, subcutaneous tissue, supraspinous and interspinous ligaments. Then a narrow (24–29G) pencil-point needle is advanced until a click is felt, indicating penetration of the dura. Free flow of cerebrospinal fluid (when the stylet is removed) confirms correct placement, and 2–3 ml 0.5% bupivacaine is injected. The patient is then placed supine and monitoring continued, as onset of sympathetic, motor, and sensory block is rapid (2–5 min). Block height and adequacy can be tested by pinprick and loss of temperature sensation. An intrathecal catheter can be sited for continuous spinal anesthesia.

Complications of this procedure include hypotension, urinary retention and bradycardia. The incidence of post-dural puncture headache is reduced by use of narrow-gauge pencil-point spinal needles. Neurological complications are extremely rare, and may be due to infection, nerve root damage, prolonged hypotension or spinal hematoma.

Absolute contraindications to this procedure include local sepsis, patient refusal, deranged clotting and full therapeutic anticoagulation. Antiplatelet therapy, neurological disease and aortic or mitral stenosis (profound hypotension can occur due to sympathetic blockade) are relative contra-indications.

Caudal Analgesia

This provides epidural analgesia below the level of the umbilicus for 4–8 h. The patient is placed in the lateral position with legs flexed at the hip. The sacral hiatus forms an equilateral triangle

TABLE 15.1. Medical therapy used in urological analgesia.

Name	Dose	Mode of action	Main side effects	Important interactions and contraindications
Paracetamol (acetaminophen)	1 g 4–6 h to max. 4 g/24 h PO/IV	Inhibits impulse generation in bradykinin-sensitive chemoreceptors; antipyretic	Idiosyncratic GI, skin disturbances, thrombocytopenia	Caution in renal or hepatic impairment
NSAIDS (ibuprofen, diclofenac)	1.2–1.8 g daily to max. 2.4 g 150 mg/24 h in divided doses PO/IM/IV	Inhibits cyclo-oxygenase formation of prostaglandins and thromboxanes; anti-inflammatory and antipyretic	Hypersensitivity, bronchospasm, GI discomfort and ulceration, inhibition of platelet aggregation	Caution in renal, hepatic or cardiac impairment
Codeine/Dihydro-codeine	30–60 mg 4–6 h PO/IM/IV	Opioid receptor agonist; variable metabolism to morphine; antitussive, anorexia	Nausea, vomiting, dizziness, constipation	Reduce dose in renal failure
Tramadol	50–100 mg to max. 400 mg daily PO/IM/IV	Opioid receptor agonist, inhibits noradrenaline and serotonin reuptake	Nausea, dizziness, sedation, acute respiratory depression	Caution in renal or hepatic failure; reduce dose
Morphine	5–20 mg PO; 15–30 mg PR; 0.1–0.2 mg/kg SC/IM; 0.05–0.1 mg/kg IV 4 h; PCA	Opioid receptor agonist, decreases membrane excitability	Nausea, vomiting, constipation, respiratory depression, euphoria, sedation, histamine release (hypotension, bronchoconstriction)	Reduce dose in renal and hepatic failure; tolerance and dependence may occur

Drug	Dose	Mechanism	Side effects/Toxicity	Notes
Diamorphine	5–10 mg PO/SC/IM; 2.5–5 mg IV	Prodrug of morphine, faster onset	As morphine	As morphine
Oxycodone	5 mg PO/SC initially to max 400 mg daily; 1–10 mg IV 4 h	As morphine	As morphine	As morphine
Fentanyl	0.5–1 μg/kg/min	Context sensitive narcotic analgesic	As morphine	As morphine
Lidocaine (lignocaine)	3 mg/kg plain, 7 mg/kg with 1:200,000 adrenaline	Reversible sodium channel blockade preventing impulse conduction; antiarrhythmic	Toxicity (overdose/IV administration) causing dizziness, seizures, arrhythmias, coma, and cardiac arrest, allergy.	Clearance reduced in cardiac and renal failure
Bupivacaine (levobupivacaine)	2 mg/kg plain or with adrenaline	As lidocaine	As lidocaine; marked cardiotoxicity	As lidocaine
Amitriptyline	10–25 mg PO increasing to 75 mg daily	Potentiate amines in CNS; sedative and antidepressant	Anticholinergic, cardiovascular, CNS, GI and hematological disturbances	Potentiates cardiovascular effects of adrenaline, Caution in those with recent MI and those with arrhythmias
Gabapentin	300 mg PO, increasing to 1.8 g daily	May bind to calcium channels in CNS	CNS, hematological and liver disturbances, diarrhea, dyspepsia, dry mouth, nausea	Reduce dose in elderly, diabetes and renal failure

with the posterior superior iliac spines. The sacral hiatus itself is a triangle formed by the sacral coruna and the fourth sacral vertebra and is covered by the sacrococcygeal membrane. A small stab incision is made midway between the sacral coruna and a 21G needle or 20G IV cannula is inserted at a 60° angle to the skin. A click is felt as the needle penetrates the sacrococcygeal membrane. The needle should be flattened and then advanced 1–2 mm, progressing easily. Bupivacaine is injected in a dose of 20–25 ml of 0.125–0.5% to a maximum of 2 mg/kg (0.5–1.0 mg/kg bupivacaine in children, depending on desired block height), aspirating frequently for blood or cerebrospinal fluid. Opioids can extend the duration of the block, but increase the risk of urinary retention and must be preservative-free.

Adrenaline has been implicated in cases of spinal ischemia and should be avoided. Potential side effects include motor block, urinary retention, hypotension, inadvertent dural puncture and intravascular injection.

Dorsal Penile Nerve Block

This is mainly performed for circumcision or other penile procedures such as meatoplasty, frenuloplasty or preputioplasty. A dorsal penile nerve block is performed with a mixture of 10 ml of 1% Lidocaine (short acting for the procedure) and 10 ml of 0.5% Bupivacaine (long acting for postoperative pain relief). The under surface of the pubic symphysis is palpated at the base of the penis. A needle is introduced vertically through Buck's fascia and the anesthetic agent is infiltrated under the symphysis pubis slightly laterally on both sides to block the dorsal nerves. Sensory sparing of the frenulum and ventral surface may occur which necessitate local anesthetic infiltration of the subcutaneous tissue at the base of the penis ventrally.

An alternative, but equally efficacious penile block can be performed using the "ring block" technique. It is straightforward technique, and is broadly similar to the technique used on other extremities, such as fingers, for reduction of fractures. Again, 10 ml 1% Lidocaine and 10 ml of 0.5% Bupivacaine are circumferentially infiltrated around the base of the penis into the loose subcutaneous connective tissues.

In overweight patients it can be difficult to accurately infiltrate under the symphysis pubis, due to increasing prepubic fat pad depth. The surgeon may need to push the prepubic fat pad down and pulling the penis up to provide an injection site sufficiently far away from the foreskin. If it fails to produce anesthesia then a "ring block" may be more appropriate [2].

Spermatic Cord Block

This is often used to provide intra-scrotal anesthesia for hydrocoele repair. It is important to remember that scrotal skin is separately innervated, and so must be additionally infiltrated to provide anesthesia. It is the authors experience that it is helpful to tell patients that they will feel normal skin sensation in the scrotal skin away from the infiltrated site, and that they will still feel movement or "pulling" during the procedure. This is because the local anesthetic agent will block the finer unmyelinated pain conduction nerves, but not the thicker myelinated proprioception fibers.

The simplest technique is to grasp the cord on each side (as it exits from the superficial inguinal ring to enter the scrotal neck). Local anesthesia can be provided with 10–20 ml of 0.5% bupivacaine. It is crucial not to infiltrate the cord at a point too far distal to the superficial ring, as this makes subsequent identification of the vas deferens, during surgery, extremely challenging, increasing the risk of iatrogenic injury to this structure.

Inguino-Scrotal Surgery

It is possible to perform inguino-scrotal procedures under local anesthesia, and this has been shown by the increasing number of inguinal hernia cases and hydrocele surgeries being undertaken with this technique.

The ilio-inguinal nerve is blocked by inserting the needle vertically 1 cm medial to the anterior superior iliac spine and then, after it has been felt to pass through the external oblique fascia, the local anesthetic agent is injected. This may be a technically difficult technique to perform successfully, with variable outcomes, and hence it is often more practical to simply infiltrate the site of the proposed incision at skin and subcutaneous tissue level, and then to infiltrate the cord at the deep inguinal ring once the surgical wound is appropriately exposed. Additional local anesthetic can be used if there are still areas of discomfort.

Transrectal Ultrasound (TRUS) Guided Prostate Biopsies

Local anesthesia significantly reduces pain and discomfort, during this diagnostic procedure. The initial paper to describe the use of local anesthetic infiltration for this procedure was by Nash et al. [3] in a series of 64 patients, in whom one side of prostate had been injected with either 5 ml of Saline or 1% Lidocaine just lateral to the junction of the seminal vesicles and the prostate on both sides (guided by the TRUS). In this study both groups had lower pain scores for the injected sides, but the reduction for Lidocaine was significantly better than that for saline [3]. Local infiltration of anesthesia in TRUS-guided prostate biopsies was later modified by Soloway et al., who incorporated two further injections on each side at the mid-portion of the prostate on the lateral aspect, and at the apex. Only one of his series of 50 men had significant discomfort [4].

Flexible Cystoscopy

This diagnostic procedure is used very commonly in urological practice, to investigate hematuria or lower urinary tract symptoms, as well as for following up patients with known bladder cancer. Traditionally flexible cystoscopy is performed under local anesthaesia which consists of urethral instillation with local anesthetic gel (Instillagel™). Instillagel™ is a mixture of 2% lidocaine and antiseptics and is available in 11 ml specially designed sterile syringes [5].

Extracorporeal Shock-Wave Lithotripsy

This is a common non-invasive method used for the treatment of renal stones less than 2 cm. Pain during the procedure is usually caused by the effect of the acoustic shock waves on the stone which can result in bruising of the kidney. In addition, subsequent passage of stone fragments down the ureter can cause renal colic-like symptoms. Simple analgesics (such as NSAIDs) given before or during the procedure can achieve good pain control.

In some centers, IV infusion of fentanyl (such as sufentanil and remifentanil) can be used for control of severe pain during the procedure although it is a highly skilled technique and requires the involvement of an anesthetist [6]. Patients who develop severe pain and fever after the procedure should be properly investigated with abdominal CT scan to exclude perinephric hematoma or hydronephrosis due to lower ureteric obstruction by stone fragments.

Postoperative Analgesia

Good postoperative pain control can alleviate the patient's distress, reduce postoperative complications and speed recovery and discharge. The choice of postoperative analgesia depends on the nature and duration of the surgery, anesthetic technique used, the staff and equipment available, and patient factors such as co morbidities and patient's perception of pain (Table 15.2). The World Health Organisation Pain Ladder [7] was originally developed as a method of managing cancer pain, and is now widely used in all pain management. The principle is to start at the bottom of the ladder, moving up if pain persists.

Regional anesthetic techniques can also be used including topical and local anesthetics infiltration, peripheral nerve block and the use of spinal and epidural anesthesia.

Patient-Controlled Analgesia (PCA)

Patient-controlled analgesia (PCA) enables patients to administer their own postoperative analgesia to suit their

TABLE 15.2.   Analgesia used for postoperative pain control.

Step 1: Mild pain	Nonopioid analgesic (aspirin, paracetamol, NSAIDS)
	± Adjuvants (steroids, antidepressants, anticonvulsants, exercise, psychological support, complimentary therapy)
Step 2: Moderate pain	Weak opioid analgesic (tramadol, codeine, dihydrocodeine)
	± Nonopioid analgesic
	± Adjuvants
Step 3: Severe pain	Strong opioid analgesic (morphine, diamorphine, oxycodone)
	± Nonopioid analgesic
	± Adjuvants

requirements. It can be administered by oral, inhalational, subcutaneous, and epidural routes, but the commonest form delivers a predetermined dose of opioid via the intravenous route using a programmed pump. The patient presses a button when in pain, and a small bolus dose of opioid (usually morphine) is delivered. This triggers a preprogrammed lockout period, during which no further analgesia can be delivered despite further demands from the patient. Overdose is also prevented by the sedative effect of morphine, so the patient will not demand any further doses until their level of the drug is reduced. A commonly used regime is 1 mg bolus dose of morphine with a 5-min lockout. Loading doses and background infusions can be programmed, but are less commonly used. Complications are related to the drug used, mechanical problems, such as siphoning, staff and patient education in the use of the device. Concurrent use of nonopioid analgesics, such as regular paracetamol and NSAID, will act synergistically and reduce the total amount of morphine required.

Emergency Management of Renal (Ureteric) Colic

Renal colic is characterized by sudden sharp pain in the flank. It radiates down (according to the site of stone impaction) to the groin, the testicle in males and the labia in females in distal ureteric stones. Stones impacted in the vesico-ureteric junction cause pain at the tip of the penis and UTI-like symptoms like frequency, urgency and dysuria. Typically patients with renal colic will be moving around and unable to lie still due to the intensity of pain.

Pain relief is the primary objective in renal colic. The current guidelines suggest that starting patients on NSAIDs (such as diclofenac) is associated with better pain control and less side effects [8, 9]. Patients with persistent pain following NSAID administration should be offered other opioid analgesics such as morphine. An antiemetic is usually given concomitantly to overcome the nausea and vomiting associated with these drugs.

Finally, medical expulsive therapy is considered efficacious and can be recommended, specifically in patients with ureteric stones <10 mm, whose symptoms are controlled, who are not septic, and who have adequate renal reserve. With regard to specific medical treatment, a published meta-analysis has shown that 29% more patients receiving α blocker therapy Tamsulosin, passed their stones than did controls, a difference that was statistically significant [8].

Key points

1. An understanding of the pain control ladder is essential to adequately manage painful urological conditions with minimal side effects.
2. Appropriate knowledge of relevant anatomy and local anesthetic drugs enables the urologist to perform a variety of minor procedures under local anesthesia.
3. Procedures performed under local anesthesia will avoid risks of general anesthesia and will ensure early recovery.
4. Adequate postoperative pain relief in patients with major urological interventions is essential for prompt recovery.
5. The urological patient should be able to decide about the preferred mode of pain relief postoperatively. This is only done after careful discussion with anesthetist and the urologist.

References

1. International Association for the study of pain (1979) Pain terms: a list with definitions and notes on usage. Recommended by the IASP Subcommittee on Taxonomy. Pain 6(3):249
2. Lander J, Brady-Fryer B, Metcalfe J et al (1997) Comparison of ring block, dorsal penile nerve block, and topical anesthesia for neonatal circumcision: a randomized controlled trial. JAMA 278(24):2157–2162
3. Nash PA, Bruce JE, Indudhara R, Shinohara K (1996) Transrectal ultrasound guided prostatic nerve blockade eases systematic needle biopsy of the prostate. J Urol 155(2):607–609
4. Soloway MS, Öbek C (2000) Periprostatic local anaesthesia before ultrasound-guided TRUS biopsy. J Urol 163:172–173
5. Brekkan E, Ehrnebo M, Malmström PU, Norlén BJ, Wirbrant A (1991) A controlled study of low and high volume anesthetic jelly as a lubricant and pain reliever during cystoscopy. J Urol 146(1):24–27
6. Beloeil H, Corsia G, Coriat P, Riou B (2002) Remifentanil compared with sufentanil during extra-corporeal shock wave lithotripsy with spontaneous ventilation: a double-blind, randomized study. Br J Anaesth 89(4):567–570
7. WHO's pain ladder. World Health Organisation 74 (1986) URL http://www.who.int/cancer/palliative/painladder/en/
8. Tiselius HG, Ackermann D, Alken P et al (2007) Guidelines in urolithiasis. European association of urology guidelines. URL http://www.uroweb.org/nc/professional-resources/guidelines/online/
9. Holdgate A, Pollock T (2005) Nonsteroidal anti-inflammatory drugs (NSAIDs) versus opioids for acute renal colic. Cochrane Database Syst Rev 18(2):CD004137

Chapter 16
Alternative or Complementary Treatments in Urology

Charlotte L. Foley, Sergiy Tadtayev, and Tamsin J. Greenwell

Introduction

Alternative medicine encompasses any healing practice that falls outside the realm of conventional medicine. When applied in conjunction with conventional treatments, it becomes "Complementary medicine." In the West, alternative medicine includes aromatherapy, Alexander technique, reflexology, hypnotherapy, acupuncture, homeopathy, meditation, biofeedback, yoga, Shiatsu, chiropractics, herbalism, traditional Chinese medicine and many more. Clearly, in other parts of the world, some such practices are mainstream techniques. The definition of alternative medicine therefore depends on context.

Alternative medicine has been variably embraced by conventional medical practitioners. The use of herbal extracts (phytotherapy) for benign prostatic hyperplasia (BPH) is widespread in Europe, and even reimbursed by health insurers in Germany, while the same treatments are considered alternative in the UK and USA. A popularly

C.L. Foley (✉)
Department of Urology, Whipps Cross University Hospital, London, UK
e-mail: charlotte.foley@whippsx.nhs.uk

I.S. Shergill et al. (eds.), *Medical Therapy in Urology*,
DOI 10.1007/978-1-84882-704-2_16,
© Springer-Verlag London Limited 2010

stated distinction is that most alternative treatments have not been submitted to rigorous, unbiased evaluation in randomized controlled trials (RCTs). This accusation may be leveled at many well-established conventional treatments too, but the current evidence for many alternative practices is weak, nonexistent, or negative. There are some exceptions, such as certain herbs (e.g., Cranberry for urinary tract infection, UTI) and acupuncture, and it is notable that these more proven alternative treatments have been brought into standard practice in some centers. However, it is unlikely that many alternative interventions will be similarly accepted until they prove themselves in clinical trials.

The concern with herbal preparations is that they are held to less stringent manufacturing and quality control procedures than pharmaceuticals. This results in considerable variability in the concentrations of active ingredients, ranging from 0 to 95% in an analysis of 27 different saw palmetto products. One herbal extract contains many (often uncharacterized) active chemicals with various actions, some of which may be undesirable. In fact, many preparations are combinations of plants – which are not only patentable, but also more marketable. PC-Spes, for example, contained extracts from eight traditional Chinese medicine herbs and showed promise in the treatment of prostate cancer. It was withdrawn in 2002, owing to quality control concerns and reported contamination with warfarin, indomethacin and diethylstilbesterol. Such cautionary tales demonstrate both the potential of phytotherapies and the need for their careful evaluation.

Public acceptance of alternative medicine is far more enthusiastic. In 1990, 34% of Americans had used alternative medicine that year, with this figure rising to 42% in 1997. It is quite likely that many urological patients have tried alternative medicines. However, only about 40% of patients report such use to their physician.

Medical Therapies using Alternative or Complementary Treatments for Urological Conditions

Benign Prostatic Hyperplasia

Saw Palmetto

The best investigated prostate phytotherapy is an extract of saw palmetto or American dwarf palm berries (*Serenoa repens*, see Table 16.1). A systematic review of 18 studies involving 2,900 patients found significant though modest improvements in overall symptom score (1.41 points), peak flow rate (1.93 ml/s), and nocturia (0.76 episodes/night) when compared with placebo. The conclusion was that Saw palmetto provided symptom improvements comparable with finasteride, with fewer adverse events.

A meta-analysis of trials using a standardized preparation (Permixon®) reported significant (and again modest) improvements in maximum flow rates and nocturia. Saw palmetto reduced symptom scores by 4.78 points, which compares well with conventional drugs. However, placebo effects are often impressive in short-term BPH trials, and placebo showed a 4.54 point reduction, which was not significantly different to saw palmetto. Thus, phytotherapies often perform better in trials against conventional medical treatments than against placebo. Two other 6-month RCTs found no benefit, and nor did a rigorous year-long RCT of 225 BPH patients for symptom score, peak flow rate, prostate size, residual urine volume, quality of life, or prostate-specific antigen (PSA) levels.

African Plum Tree

Extracts from the bark of the African plum tree (*Pygeum africanum* and *Prunus africanum*) are also active in the prostate (Table 16.1). A Cochrane meta-analysis of 18 tri-

TABLE 16.1.   Phytotherapies used in LUTS/benign prostatic hyperplasia (BPH).

Name	Postulated mode of action	Dose	Main side effects	Important interactions and contraindications
Saw palmetto	Antiandrogenic, proliferative, inhibit prolactin growth factor and 5-alpha reductase, antiestrogenic, anti-inflammatory	160 mg daily (as Permixon®)	Nausea, abdominal pain, diarrhea, alteration in taste, urticaria	Pre-existing serious abdominal disorders
African plum tree	Growth factor inhibition, anti-inflammatory, reduce detrusor contractility, reduce luteinizing hormone, testosterone, and prolactin	50 mg twice daily	Diarrhea, constipation, dizziness, headache	None reported
African star grass	Anti-inflammatory, proapoptotic, antiproliferative	60 mg (as Harzol®) 65 mg (as Azuprostat®) daily	Diarrhea, constipation	Hyperglycemia, Inhibition of cytochrome p450
Pumpkin seeds	Anti-inflammatory, Antiandrogen	30 g or 160 mg thrice daily as pumpkin seed oil	None reported	Possibly increases warfarin effect (though implicated as a component of a combination phytotherapy)
Rye grass pollen	Antiandrogenic, reduce urethral resistance, increase detrusor contraction, alpha-blocker actions	126 mg twice daily	Nausea	None reported
Stinging nettle	Anti-inflammatory, antiproliferative	240 mg nettle root extract daily	Nausea, rash, sweating, diarrhea	Hypertension, Hyperglycemia

Note: Mechanisms of action are in general poorly understood, with minimal in vivo conformation of in vitro effects als involving 1,562 men showed a twofold improvement in symptom scores, a 23% increase in flow rates, and a 19% reduction in nocturia. Adverse effects were mild. A review of published trials using a standardized *P africanum* preparation (Tadenan®) identified 2,262 patients across many small, short trials. None of them met the standard recommended by the International Consultation Conferences on BPH, and as such, the data on *P africanum*'s efficacy are inconclusive.

South African Stargrass

Two preparations of South African stargrass (*Hypoxis rooperi*), which is rich in beta-sitosterol and other sterols, have been studied. The Harzol® trial randomized 200 patients to Harzol® or placebo, showing substantial and significant improvements when compared with placebo in symptom score (7.3 vs. 2.3 points) and peak flow rate (5.2 vs. 1.1 ml/s). The Azuprostat® trial randomized 177 patients to Azuprostat® or placebo and showed similarly impressive, significant results (8.3 vs. 2.8 symptom score points, 8.8 vs. 4.4 ml/s in peak flow). These results exceed most conventional BPH drug effects and approach those of surgery. However, the placebo group also performed unusually well, and though mean patient age was 65, the peak flow rate in the treatment group was surprisingly high at 19.4 ml/s, which raises questions of validity.

Pumpkin Seed

Pumpkin seeds (*Cucurbita pepo*) are popular in Germany. Few trials have evaluated them. However, a 1-year RCT of 476 patients reported impressive symptom score improvements of 6.8 points, which was a significant 1.2 points better than placebo (which also performed moderately well).

Rye Pollen

An extract of rye grass pollen (*Secale cereale*) called cernilton was subjected to a Cochrane review. Evidence from 440 men in four trials suggested some effect on self-rated improvement and nocturia, but none in flow rate, residual urine, or prostate size over placebo, though withdrawal rates were low at 4.8%. The Cochrane authors reported "modest" effects; however, the Oxford evidence-based healthcare journal, Bandolier, concluded no evidence of any benefit.

Stinging Nettle

A stinging nettle (*Urtica dioica*) preparation Prostagutt® was as effective as finasteride in a year-long RCT involving 489 patients. It achieved dramatic improvements in symptom score (4.8–7.5 points) and in peak urinary flow (2–3 ml/s). An 18-month placebo-controlled cross-over study on 620 men reported similar and significant magnitudes of effect across all usual outcome measures. However, further trials are necessary before this promising agent can be recommended.

   Other phytotherapies for BPH have been evaluated even less. Results within and between trials are often mixed, and none have the scale and longevity of conventional BPH treatments.

Prostate Cancer

Vitamin E

Cancer patients in particular are frequent adopters of complementary medicine. Patients on active surveillance are keen to pursue lifestyle and dietary measures that will influence the progression of their disease, while increasing awareness of men's health issues has raised interest in preventative measures.

   The antioxidant vitamin E has been evaluated for various health benefits in large population studies. The 6-year, 29,133 patient ATBC study suggested that male smokers given 50 mg vitamin E daily had a significantly (32%) lower incidence of prostate cancer than those on placebo. However, the 7-year HOPE Trial found that vitamin E did not reduce the incidence of prostate cancer, total cancer, or major cardiovascular events. The ongoing SELECT trial (Selenium and vitamin E cancer prevention trial) will evaluate the effect of 200 mcg selenium, 400 mg vitamin E, both, or placebo on prostate cancer incidence in >35,000 men. Follow-up will be for 12 years, but a press release issued in October 2008 reported an interim analysis suggesting that selenium and vitamin E did not prevent prostate cancer, and participants were asked to stop their supplements. Furthermore, two nonstatistically significant trends require further evaluation: slightly more cases of prostate cancer occurred in men taking vitamin E alone, and there were slightly more cases of diabetes in those taking only selenium. Completion of follow-up and further analysis will ensue, but vitamin E cannot currently be recommended.

Selenium

The trace element selenium was implicated when reduced cancer risk was correlated with higher soil selenium levels. A study on prevention of nonmelanoma skin cancer identified a reduction in prostate cancer incidence as a secondary endpoint. The SELECT trial was designed to investigate this further, but recent events suggest that selenium is not preventative (see Vitamin E above).

Lycopene

Lycopene is found in tomatoes, lychees, and pink grapefruit. The effect of dietary or supplemental lycopene on serum PSA levels has been evaluated in a number of patient groups with conflicting results. Three weeks of lycopene prior to radical prostatectomy in 26 patients with localized cancer was associated with a drop in PSA when compared with a rise in the untreated group. Other pathological parameters also seemed more favorable, but numbers were too small to allow firm conclusions. Conversely, a year-long trial on patients with biochemical relapse showed no effect on PSA progression, but adding lycopene to orchidectomy in 54 men with advanced disease produced a more consistent serum PSA reduction and improved bone pain, lower urinary tract symptoms, and survival.

Pomegranate Juice

A single uncontrolled trial of pomegranate juice in 48 men with rising PSA levels after definitive local therapy showed a significant reduction in PSA doubling time. Demand for pomegranate juice rocketed 250% after these results were reported in the popular press. However, further confirmatory trials are needed and drug interactions are possible (Table 16.2).

Chronic Prostatitis

Chronic prostatitis can have a greatly deleterious effect on quality of life, and patients living with this condition learn to cope with unpredictable and chronic pain, lower urinary tract symptoms, and sexual problems. Often, conventional treatments will have had disappointing outcomes, so alternative medicine offers another approach, particularly for those with type III prostatitis/chronic pelvic pain syndrome.

Quercetin

This is a bioflavinoid found in citrus fruit, apples, greens, and onions among others with anti-inflammatory and antioxidant properties – both processes implicated in the etiology of chronic prostatitis. A 1-month RCT of 30 patients showed that 67% had a clinically significant response in the treatment arm when compared with 20% for placebo. Prostaglandin and leukocyte levels fell in prostatic secretions while endorphins rose. Reported side effects included some nausea and tingling. Quercetin also inhibits CYP3A resulting in drug interactions and may block the action of quinolone antibiotics.

Bladder Pain Syndrome/Interstitial Cystitis (BPS/IC)

Similar motivations and approaches apply to painful bladder syndrome; however, the lack of evidence means that no treatments can be recommended. Dietary avoidance of

TABLE 16.2.   Alternative therapies for prostate cancer.

Name	Postulated mode of action	Dose	Main side effects	Important interactions and contraindications
Vitamin E	Antioxidant effects	50 or 400 mg daily	Abdominal pain and diarrhea at doses >1 g/day	Care in those predisposed to thrombosis
Selenium	Antioxidant effects	200 mcg daily	Nausea, vomiting, abdominal pain Toxic at doses >900 mcg/day	Ascorbic acid, cisplatin, oral corticosteroid, and clozapine can reduce selenium effects
Lycopene	Antiproliferative, anti-oxidant, proapoptotic	2–30 mg daily	None reported	Dietary lipids enhance bio-availability
Pomegran-ate juice	Antioxidant, proapop-totic, antibacterial	8 oz of juice daily	None reported	Cytochrome CYP3A inhibition similar to that of grapefruit juice Enhancement of antistaphy-lococcal antibiotic activity

exacerbating foods is widely practised, but often individualized. Successes in series of patients have been reported for acupuncture (79% > 50% improvement), myofascial trigger point release (70% improvement), transvaginal massage, and quercetin (significant symptom score improvement).

Urinary Tract infection

Cranberry Juice

There is good evidence that cranberry juice prevents and may treat UTIs in susceptible women, but not in neuropathic patients or children. Cranberry and blueberry juices contain proanthocyanidins that interfere with *E. coli* adherence to the urothelium. Trials used 200–750 ml of cranberry juice, but the actual cranberry content of preparations can vary. Cranberry juice halved the number of UTIs representing a "number needed to treat" of 14 (or 8 if only trials over 6 months are considered). However, dropout rates were approximately 40% and high cranberry juice intake has been reported to interact with warfarin.

Peyronie's Disease

This poorly understood, chronic condition has many treatments with scant evidence for their efficacy. Vitamin E (400 IU/day) is a common treatment with few positive trial outcomes, but at least does no harm. Acetyl-L-Carnitine has been found to be superior to tamoxifen in one study. It achieved 92% pain reduction and inhibition of disease progression and seven degrees of penile straightening.

Erectile Dysfunction

In no other area of urology are there more herbal remedies available, with the least likelihood of any proven efficacy. It is likely that herbal extracts do contain erectogenic compounds, and combined with the 25–50% placebo effect seen in conventional trials, the "herbal viagra" market remains healthy. However, the unregulated nature of these products was demonstrated in an analysis, which found treatment levels of sildenafil and tadalafil in only two of seven internet-bought products, with the accompanying serious drug interaction risks.

Korean Red Ginseng

Korean Red or Panax Ginseng contains ginsenosides, which increase nitric oxide release, thereby causing smooth muscle relaxation. This herbal preparation has been evaluated in a number of clinical trials, performing significantly better than placebo and achieving a 60–66% response rates.

Conclusions

At worst, alternative therapies defraud unwell patients with harmful interventions; at best they are therapies with superior efficacy to current drugs yet fewer side effects, and often in disease areas where conventional treatments have little to offer. Evidence based medicine will help discriminate between therapies, so appropriately and carefully designed trials of each treatment should be welcomed by all practitioners.

Key Points

1. The use of complementary/alternative medicine is widespread, and may not be divulged by patients, unless the information is directly requested.
2. Herbal preparations may have unpredictable concentrations of active ingredients, contaminants, and drug interactions.
3. Evidence is insufficient to allow recommendation of most alternative therapies except cranberry for UTI, though there are promising treatments worthy of further study.

4. Studies are hampered by variable dosing, large placebo responses in chronic urological diseases, and the difficulty of blinding some active treatments.
5. Formal randomized-controlled studies are needed before conventional medicine can recommend alternative treatments.

Further Reading

1. Eisenberg DM, Davis RB, Ettner SL (1998) Trends in alternative medicine use in the United States 1990–1997. JAMA 280:1569–1575
2. Izzo AA, Ernst E (2001) Interactions between herbal medicines and prescribed drugs: a systematic review. Drugs 61:2163–2175
3. Dreikorn K (2002) The role of phytotherapy in treating lower urinary tract symptoms and benign prostatic hyperplasia. World J Urol 19:426–435
4. Bent S, Kane C, Shinohara K, Neuhaus J, Hudes ES, Goldberg H, Avins AL (2006) Saw palmetto for benign prostatic hyperplasia. N Engl J Med 354:557–566
5. Moyad MA, Barada JH, Lue TF, Mulhall JP, Goldstein I, Fawzy A (2004) Sexual medicine society nutraceutical committee. Prevention and treatment of erectile dysfunction using lifestyle changes and dietary supplements: what works and what is worthless, part II. Urol Clin North Am 31:259–273
6. Ernst E (2007) Herbal medicines: balancing benefits and risks. Novartis Found Symp 282:154–167

Index